HARDEN THE F*CK UP

HARDEN THE F*CK UP

No-Nonsense Fitness insights
from the **World's Leading Experts**
to make you *Harder to Kill*

DAVE MORROW

Library and Archives Canada Cataloguing in Publication
Morrow, Dave, author
Harden the Fuck Up / Dave Morrow

Issued in print and electronic formats.
ISBN: 978-1-998501-30-4 (paperback)
ISBN: 978-1-998501-31-1 (ebook)

Cover Design: Pablo Javier Herrera
Interior Design: Winston S. Prescott

Double Dagger Books Ltd.
Toronto, Ontario, Canada
www.doubledagger.ca

TABLE OF CONTENTS

This book is dedicated to Stephanie, Xavier and Olivia. You've been the bedrock of my recovery. I'm forever grateful for your love, humor and light you bring to my life everyday. Abracadabra.

FOREWORD

At the young age of 17, I made a decision that would shape the course of my life—I joined the United States Marine Corps. Back then, my understanding of the world was limited. My biggest concerns were what my favorite TV show was and where I wanted to eat on a Friday night with my family. The concept of being "Hard to Kill" was something I associated with a Seagal movie, not a way of life.

But time and experience have a way of reshaping our understanding. After leaving the Marines and surviving a harrowing combat deployment to Iraq, I realized that being "Hard to Kill" had little to do with the rigorous physical training I received in bootcamp or the tactical skills honed in follow-on schools. It was about something much deeper—mental acuity and mindfulness. It was about becoming a warrior in the garden.

As the echoes of rifle fire, mortars, and cannons have faded for many of us, the resilience required today is more demanding than what was needed on the battlefield. The battles we face now—within ourselves and our society—require us to choose response over reaction, empathy over apathy, and vigilance over carelessness. These disciplines are the pillars of resilience, a testament to the journey that continues long after the dust of combat has settled.

Being hard to kill is not just about physical strength; it's about the strength of character and spirit. Just like our physical muscles, these qualities must be nurtured and developed over time. As they are tested, they grow, forming the calluses only experience can provide. Through this process, we harden our minds, bodies, and spirits, enriching our understanding of what it truly means to be healthy—both physically and mentally.

In a world that increasingly demands a robust digital presence and online persona, it's crucial to stay grounded in our physical and mental health. We must recognize where we are vulnerable and where we are strong, identify areas for improvement, and learn to let go of what no longer serves us. The human condition requires active participation. The question is, how do you show up?

Between the COVID-19 pandemic and the fall of Kabul, I witnessed just how fragile our mental health can be—both within the US military and the civilian community. The shock, shame, and hopelessness that gripped so many Americans were heartbreaking. Mental health emergencies skyrocketed, and the US Veterans Affairs took a proactive approach for the first time, offering healthcare solutions that met veterans where they were, saving countless lives in the process.

To truly grasp the gravity of the situation, consider this: since 2001, over 150,000 veterans have taken their own lives—a staggering figure compared to the 68,000 combat deaths in all wars fought since Vietnam. The war didn't end for these veterans; it followed them home, where the battles continued long after the conflict had ended.

Isolation and withdrawal are the largest contributors to suicidal behavior, but they are not insurmountable. We can combat them by advocating for healthier, more inclusive lifestyles. Our health—both mental and physical—is one of the few things we can control. But it requires active participation. It requires showing up.

And it requires us to be hard to kill—not just in body, but in mind and spirit.

Tim Jensen,
Co-Owner & Chief Brand Officer
Grunt Style, LLC

INTRODUCTION

You're soft - accept it.

You picked up this book because you feel it when you wake up and when you go to bed at night. There's a nagging feeling that you're not doing what your body is supposed to be doing.

But what is it?

I'll tell you - Doing intentionally hard things.

Everything in our environment is telling us to relax and take it easy. You're probably reading this in a perfectly, temperature-controlled room, on a nice comfy chair with a full belly of food bought at the greatest achievement in human history - the grocery store!

It's not your fault. We're all a casualty of our collective success. Don't get me wrong, not having to constantly hunt and worry about a neighbouring tribe coming to rape and pillage my kinsmen is a net positive for us. However, we can't out-innovate our genes.

We are primal, chest-beating, meat-eating beings that have been perfectly adapted to hunt, kill, make strong interpersonal relationships and survive in every possible environment on this planet. We're incredible! Yet your complacency and acceptance of a purely "modern" lifestyle are causing you to be tired, weak and depressed. Far from incredible.

This book had to be written. Every cell in my body compels me to make myself and those around me better. Having been injured, in pain and depressed, I felt this awful pull of complacency pulling me deeper into a hole. It would whisper, "It's ok, don't struggle, why do more? There are drugs, doctors and Netflix to fix you, this is the way to happiness..."

But this is not the path to hardness and the mastery of your life. I'm not the first to come to this realization. In a response to his young colleague Epigenes, Socrates offered a response to his poor physical health:

> "The fit are healthy and strong; and many, as a consequence, save themselves decorously on the battle-field and escape all the dangers of war; many help friends and do good to their country and for this cause earn gratitude; get great glory and gain very high honours, and for this cause live henceforth a pleasanter and better life, and leave to their children better means of winning a livelihood."

It's a simple concept - everything you do in life should make you harder to kill. However, our long nap since the end of

2

the Second World War has left us soft, tired and fat. Even our warfighters, who punch Taliban maniacs in the face for freedom, can lose their way and become soft; I know, I was one of them.

Since losing my way, I've had the honour of being able to talk to some of the world's leading experts on mindset, fitness, nutrition and recovery on my Hard To Kill Podcast. This book is a summary of all the amazing knowledge I've accumulated over the last four years. During my time in the Army, I learned something very valuable – always pass info along to your buddy. So, whether you're a grizzled veteran, an Army recruit or a greasy civilian, this book will act as a field manual to establish or re-establish your hardness and make you Harder To Kill.

GETTING UP TO SPEED

I grew up in suburbia. Large parks, tons of friends and a ton of sports to play. Sure, I was chubby, but I came to compete every day. Even still, my best friends would mercilessly shame me for being fat. Kids are fucking awful eh? But, to be honest, it was coming from a place of love. I didn't know that in the moment; in between sobs I would curse their names and wish awful, hateful shit upon them and their families. But, what it did was motivate the shit out of me not to be fat anymore. By the time Grade 7 came around I was six feet tall and skinny as a broomstick. Sure, I got a huge helping hand in getting thin from my gigantic family genes, but I vowed to NEVER be fat again.

It was so bad for me growing up that I would make up excuses not to take my shirt off during our swim days in elementary school. I would get anxious around January every year since I knew the pool was coming up in June and I didn't want to show my tits to the girls I had crushes on. Every year I would say, "This year I'm going to be fit and get rid of these" but every year it was the same story. "I've got really sensitive skin because I'm Irish, so I need to wear a shirt in the pool."

That was a lie.

I remember going to the gym with my dad who was an OG, 1970's, Schwarzenegger acolyte and was my fitness idol. He showed me how to use the leg press machines and how to bench press. I would do push-ups every fricken day when I got home from school, and I'd go to the gym on weekends with him— to no avail. I would only find out about four months before writing this book that I have a medical condition called gynecomastia and no matter how much I train or cut, I'll always have these puffy boobs.

The point of all this is to say that I'm thankful for this pretty common medical issue where, just before puberty, my hormones got a little fucked up and I had a surge of estrogen that screwed up my chest and produced more fat tissue that will never go away unless I have surgery. I didn't know that. I, like everyone else, just called them "bitch tits" and that was life. I just thought: I guess I gotta train harder, eh?

I did and still do to this day. I do thousands of push-ups every year and they've never gone away even when I was at 15% body fat. Everything hard and depressing is character building, and I wouldn't be writing this book if my best friends hadn't invented a game called "Medusa tits." When we were kids and I flashed my "tits" at them, they would freeze. Freeze tag with my tits as the "freezing" agent. If you're a dude reading this,

4

and you've been dealing with the same condition, it sucks but use it to your advantage.

So now you know a little about me and my motivation to get into the fitness game. It was also a defining factor for joining the Army. Why? I needed to take my fitness to the next level and I thought: what better way to get jacked as a 19-year-old than join the Canadian Armed Forces and carry heavy shit all day and shoot guns.

ARMY LIFE

"Sir, I fucken love this shit."
- Me circa 2001, Connaught Ranges

This is what I said in week one of my basic training course during my initial interview with my platoon commander. I wasn't bullshitting either, I've never been a kiss-ass. I truly loved what I was doing; getting up early, going for runs, getting sorted out for dust on my floor. I felt like I finally found something I was good at. It felt awesome. I ended up the top candidate on that course and at the time I brushed it off as no big deal, but it defined my mindset.

I was a good, competent, fit soldier. I never was singled out for being good at anything before; I was valedictorian of my grade six class with Sheena Dubeau and Lindsay Richardson, but I don't think that counts. This one was just me, in front of all my platoon mates and soon-to-be regiment, getting a piece of paper that said, "Bro, you're good at this, keep it up!"

And I did.

Growing up, watching GI Joe and WWF religiously, I wanted

to be a soldier like Sgt Slaughter or Duke. I wanted to lead men into battle. I know I'm Canadian but man the American motivation machine of the 80s was epic. I would sing Hulk Hogan's ring entrance song at full tilt:

"I AM A REAL AMERICAN, FIGHT FOR THE RIGHTS OF EVERY MAN!"

It was infectious. I was so patriotic....for "Murica!

Either way, the stories I heard about my Grandpa Morrow fighting in the Italian campaign during World War Two and going missing in action were so fascinating to me. War was fascinating to me, and it still is. I guess it's no surprise that I liked it so much. I never really had something that I was both good at and proud of being a part of. I was so fired up

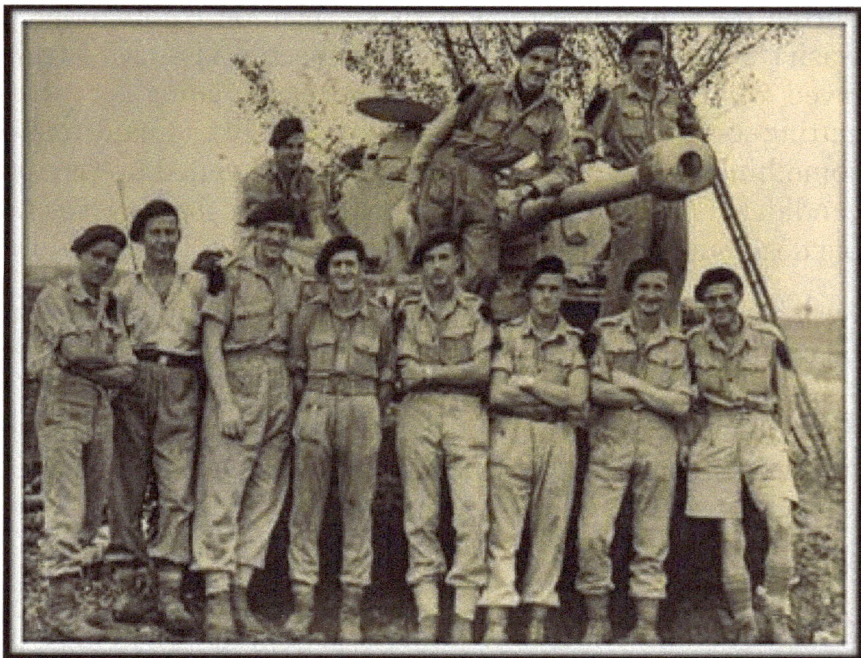

after my first summer that I went and got my first tattoo—my regiment's Brigade patch and the "grenade fired proper" of the Canadian Grenadier Guards with a nice red maple leaf inlaid behind it (the maple leaf being a required tattoo for all Canadian males to get before age 25).

I volunteered to deploy to Afghanistan in 2010. I wanted to experience the highs and lows of war and more importantly, I wanted to test myself. I had spent nearly ten years training, was a sergeant and hadn't had any operational experience. It was eating at me.

The best way to describe it would be like training to be a professional actor and learning every line of Hamlet but never actually going on stage in front of an audience. My theatre was war.

I had a very Hemingwayesque way of looking at combat. I saw it as the crucible for a man to test his mettle. I believed it to be one of humankind's most fundamental behaviours and wanted to know what it was like. I knew it was dangerous and didn't romanticize it. I knew very well that I could die or worse come home seriously maimed. This was the stone I had chosen to lift, and I was going to carry it and let its weight mould me into a better human being.

THE FALL

During my time in the Army, I considered myself a shining example of fitness. When I deployed, I was at the peak of my military career as a young sergeant in the Canadian Armed Forces. I could run my ass off, bang out a dozen pull-ups and do push-ups until my arms fell off. However, there was a lurking

7

fundamental deficiency that was like a physical ticking time bomb waiting to take me out, just like the IEDs we dodged in Afghanistan.

I built a body and career around being the "fit" guy, the competent guy, the professional guy. That all started to unravel when I got injured while on patrol in Afghanistan in 2011. No, I wasn't knee-deep in grenade pins and beating off a horde of Taliban fighters with a machine gun tripod (that has happened, but just not on my mission), I was picking up my gear and my back went "BANG".

"Oh FUCK." I said to myself, "We're under contact." But no one was reacting on my patrol. The scorching fire running up from my lower back was the result of this audible pop and then I was wondering, "Can I stand up? Can I walk? Can I get back to base?"

The last thing I wanted was to get medevaced out because I hurt my back picking up a backpack. Thank God for my massive ego. I willed myself to get back to base, dropped my gear, grabbed a handful of pills, lay down on my cot and pretended nothing happened.

At that point, I was 29 years old and in a warzone. Getting deployed to a warzone had been one of my dreams since I was a little kid. I used to play GI Joe with my best buds, I would dress up as a soldier for Halloween, and The Punisher was my favourite comic book. I visualized what combat would be like and I wanted to experience it because I felt it was and is the most visceral of all human experiences. With that said, there was no way that I was going to let a non-life-threatening injury send me home mid-way through my mission. I volunteered to go there and I wasn't about to leave.

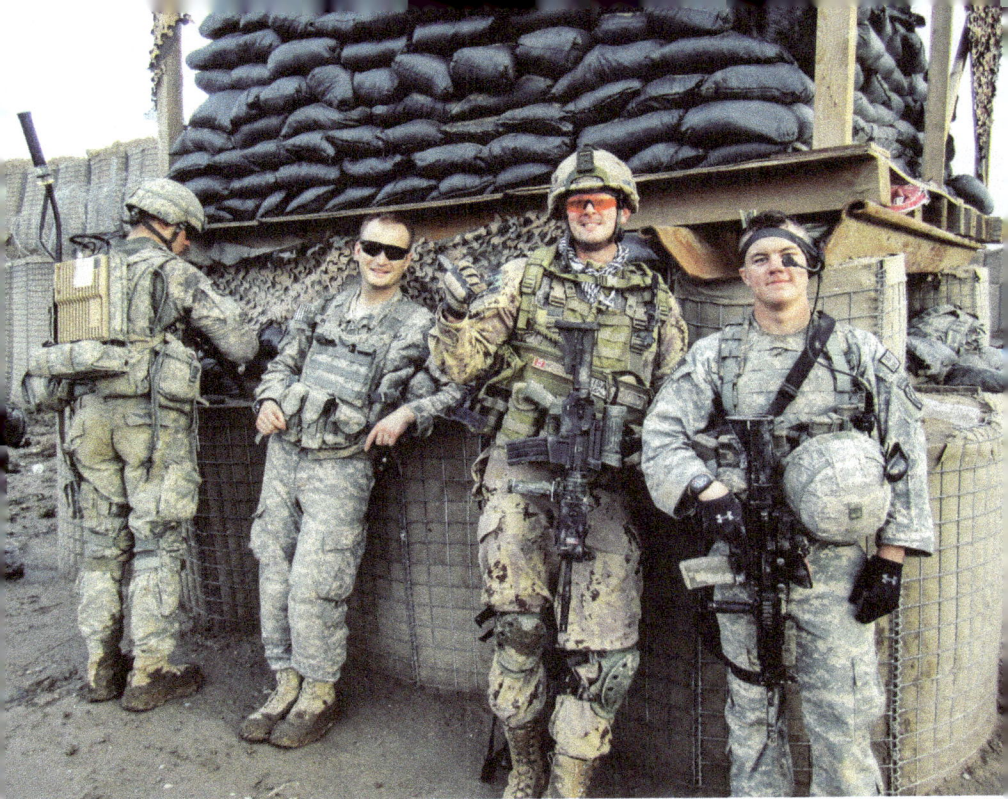

Every time I got strapped into our armoured vehicles, the compression of the safety harness would put a tremendous amount of pressure on my lower back, and I would dread any road move because of it. But I just popped more pain meds and sipped on some Ripits and kept on truckin'. I should also mention that at this point, I'd already wrenched my knee pretty badly after gracefully falling off a wall with 70 lbs of kit on. So, all in all, things were going pretty well.

Only eight years after my return home did I finally seek out help to address my wild mood swings and simmering anger that would boil over and result in me detaching from friends and family and "sorting myself out" in my basement. Things started to unravel for me right after my son was born. Admittedly, I was pretty good at maintaining the veneer of having it all together. I had a great teaching job at a high school, I was coaching football and track, and I was completing my master's degree. At around this point, I had just been released from the Forces due to my injuries and at the time, I just sloughed it off as an insignificant change. Since I was no longer "that guy" anymore, I'd moved on. Little did I know, I was simply avoiding the harsh reality that I was desperately trying to find a new identity. I was lost and trying to find my purpose again.

Well, things all took a turn for the worse when I innocuously was putting on my pants at work and "BANG" my back locked up like a bear trap. I grabbed onto my locker like Leonardo di Caprio grabbing onto the last piece of wood when the Titanic sank. And just like Leo, I sank. My buddy was in the locker room with me and offered help—but the typical, proud me said, "I'm good bro." Sweating, in agony and at a permanent 45-degree forward lean, I managed to get my broken ass up to my classroom and teach the rest of the day. Man, was I in pain. I was stuck in bed for a week after that and couldn't even go take a dump without help from my wife. This was humiliating but on top of that, I felt useless. I couldn't provide for or defend my family and I couldn't even take care of my newborn son.

I was angry. Why did this happen to me? I was fit, or so I thought.

I remember thinking while stuck in bed, "This can't be the rest of my life. I have to make a change once I can move again."

And with that determination, I sought out help.

RECOVERY

I was a member of my local Crossfit box. I liked the classes led by one of the coaches and we had a good relationship. So, I decided that I was going to invest in myself and have him help me work on the things that were a weakness of mine so that I could be functionally strong and if need be, be able to recover better from surgery.

Things got rough for me for about a year. I left my stable teaching job because I was having mini panic attacks before my students would enter the classroom. I was developing high blood pressure, didn't want to get out of bed and felt tired all the time. I got fired from a new job after three months and my world was starting to collapse in on itself.

I remember on some days only having to bring my son to daycare and it was like I had to climb Everest. Everything was hard. I would walk back home after dropping him off and choke back the tears. I was convinced I was a loser, a failure and not worthy of my family.

This was the lowest point of my life. I've never felt so completely shattered and defeated. I cried while walking home, unemployed and injured. But there was still a sliver of hope I was clinging on to. My son and my soon-to-be-born daughter were a guiding light, since providing for them—and more importantly, making them proud—was a no-fail mission of mine. So, I dug deep every day. All I wanted to do was sit in my basement and wish the world away but there was a nagging force that kept me going. That force was a new, pre-pubescent business that I had created in the wake of my last job firing.

It didn't comprise of much, but it was a reason to get up in the

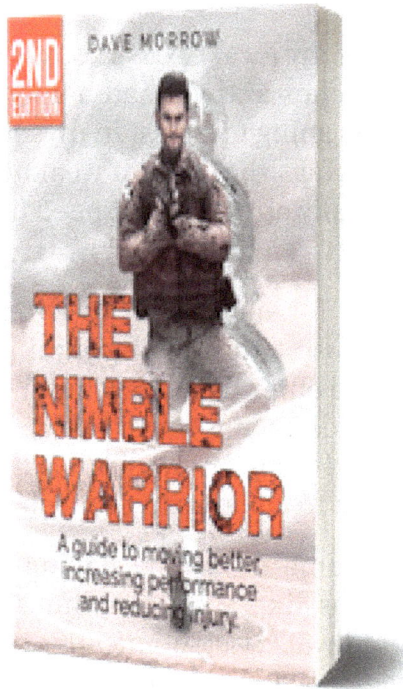

morning. I had a few coaching clients that I didn't want to let down and I was hearing from others who wanted to know more about how to prevent injuries in their Army careers. With that little spark, I decided to embark on writing a small PDF file of the exercises I used and still use to keep my back and knees in good working condition. That 4-page PDF file started to take on more and more context every day and within a month of voracious writing, I had completed my first book, The Nimble Warrior. It was like something had compelled me to write every day and it was exciting to see it take shape.

Now I coach fellow veterans, run two amazing companies that are building more solutions to veteran health and fitness problems and hosting a podcast that allows me to talk to some of the smartest people on the planet. I hope the lessons learned in the following chapters give you the clarity to define your vision, like it did for me. Next, Let's define the scope of the problem I'm trying to address.

MY MISSION

I have resolved to help one hundred thousand veterans lose two million pounds. This is important to me because, without physical health, it's very hard to be psychologically well. If we remember what Socrates said, it's also hard to do great things if you're not physically fit. Here are some sobering facts about veteran health:

Obesity: Obesity in the veteran population is higher than the national average. It is also linked to higher levels of mental health issues such as PTSD.

Suicide: Veterans are more likely to die by their own hands than by the enemy's. They are 1.5 times more likely to commit suicide compared to non-veterans.

Chronic Pain: Sixty-five percent of veterans experience chronic pain compared to fifty-six percent of non-veterans in the U.S.

Cancer: Veterans are more likely to develop cancer, in some cases up to 87% more likely than non-veterans.

Traumatic Brain Injury (TBI): A study of recent-era U.S.

veterans found that 17.3% of participants met criteria for TBI during military service, with about half reporting multiple head injuries.

BECOMING H.A.R.D. TO KILL

We can improve these statistics, but it's going to require awareness and a blueprint to make it happen. That's what I hope this book serves as. The big picture is that you need to be H.A.R.D. to kill and in harmony with your true, natural state.

H.A.R.D. stands for:

- Happy
- Aggressive
- Ready
- Disciplined

I've boiled being a healthy veteran down to a few key things that are "no-fail missions." These missions are crucial to your long-term health and longevity and are fully backed by the best science on the planet and the expert opinions of my podcast guests. At the end of this book, I'll attach a simple weekly training and habit plan you can use and adapt for the rest of your life.

Happy

This includes a massive component of finding out who you truly are. My opinion on happiness is that it isn't a pursuit but a state that arises out of satisfaction with oneself and one's actions. If you're living in shame, dealing with a victim mentality, and ruminating over issues from your service, it's going to be next to impossible, regardless of how many pharmaceuticals you take, to be "happy." If a victim mentality has taken hold of you, you need to listen to expert Mark England's words.

It's becoming increasingly evident that if you've "tried everything" to sort out your mental state, psychedelics such as ayahuasca may offer an outside-the-box solution for overcoming PTSD. Listen to the conversations with CAF veteran Ryan Carey about his healing journey.

Aggressive

This is where you need to unleash your inner warrior. It never goes away. On the contrary, going from a state of wartime readiness, where you were a lion on the savannah, to a cuddly house cat at home is very damaging to the soul. Aggressiveness, for men, is not about smashing a fist into another dude's face for stepping on your shoe; in my opinion, it's about taking action and being a leader.

You need a physically aggressive outlet to express your true self. The research is clear that a discipline like Brazilian jiu-jitsu is a very effective way for veterans to embrace their aggressiveness while building strong relationships with other warriors on the mats. Read more about it in the chapter with Dr. Gino Collura. I love Jordan Peterson's quote that embodies this very well:

> "A harmless man is not a good man. A good man is a very, very dangerous man who has that under voluntary control."

Ready

Being ready requires a sense of awareness. You don't know

what you don't know. How do you go from being unaware of looming threats and issues that can blindside you? Read, listen, watch, and learn about your environment and surroundings.

Therefore, read a minimum of 10 pages a day of anything that's not on the internet—actual books. The long-term effect of consistently reading is the creation of an always-appreciating asset that no one or government can ever take away or devalue: knowledge.

This also includes making sure your body is ready to absorb any major stress. Two of the best ways to do that are through cold exposure and breathing exercises. Cold water has been a therapy used since ancient Greece to alleviate the body's stress and dramatically improve mood. Find Brandon Powell's chapter and "Breathe Motherfucker."

Disciplined

I believe that the three most important daily habits you need to be very disciplined in are your fitness, nutrition, and sleep. I'd argue that sleep is probably the most important, especially for veterans. Eight hours is your baseline; don't complain about being better on 5 or 6 hours—it's 8. Are you going to argue with a Navy SEAL who's spent his entire professional career studying sleep? Read Dr. Kirk Parsley's chapter about sleep.

When it comes to fitness, this is a daily habit too. A minimum of 8,000 steps per day is non-negotiable. This improves longevity significantly and makes you much more resistant to type 2 diabetes and cardiovascular diseases. Doctors Brandeis, Justin, and Ovadia will all reiterate the importance of physical activity to ensure your weiner works as well as your heart.

Lastly, nutrition is where you can either pay the farm now or pay the "pharm" later. The key here is that you stay disciplined on your protein intake every day and incorporate some fasting periods every year. Cynthia Thurlow and Ben Azadi will help guide you to your new nutrition paradigm.

Veteran Health At A Glance

Obesity

Alright, here's the deal. What's the single worst disease affecting humanity today? Nope, not coronavirus, AIDS, or cancer. It's obesity. This condition is wreaking havoc because of all the subsequent diseases it causes—cancer, diabetes, high blood pressure, kidney failure, and fatty liver. The list goes on and on. You can't look around without seeing overweight people today. Being overweight over a century ago meant you had to be wealthy. Now, it's the complete opposite. The poor are the most likely to be overweight. Why is that?

A shitty science experiment.

Believe it or not, once the government gets involved in what you eat, you become a guinea pig. This is exactly what happened about 50 years ago when the U.S. government decided to enact a new law that mandated macronutrient values for foods to be considered healthy and determined which produce should be prioritized for growth. This was all based on some convincing data at the time surrounding heart disease. The concern was that we were consuming too much fat, causing the sharp increase in heart disease cases in the U.S.

Much of this research turned out to be flawed and in need of much greater peer review, but the die had been cast, and the diet-heart hypothesis was born. This hypothesis, believe it or not, has likely influenced a shit ton of your beliefs around food since you were born. Head to the chapter with Dr. Philip Ovadia for more context.

So, how does this all tie into metabolic disease? Let me explain what metabolic disease is.

Metabolic disease is the presence of any one of the following: obesity, high blood pressure, pre-diabetes, and high triglycerides. Pretty ugly stuff. I know what you're thinking, "Well, I'm skinny, bro, this ain't gonna happen to me."

This disease was brought to my attention when Dr. Peter Attia, a key figure in the medical field and a fellow Canadian, gave a great talk at TED Talks. His athletic background is impressive. He competes in ultra swim marathons, runs triathlons, and is just an overall badass. But, as he says in his TED Talk, he was becoming a victim of metabolic disease. How can a ridiculously fit doctor, who deals with sick and ill patients every day suffering from the effects of metabolic disease, be in the same category as them?

In his words,"I was disgusted with their lack of discipline. Why can't you just stop eating?"But when he realized that he was going down the same route as his patients, he knew that something was drastically wrong with what he was saying. This led him to re-examine what was considered the gold standard in nutrition and health."Eat often and eat regularly for improved performance and energy. Eat your protein bars and make sure to have a big breakfast; it's the most important meal of the day, didn't you know?"Unfortunately, this is not the case. If it were, we wouldn't be seeing obesity and diabetes rates explode across our countries. We wouldn't have child obesity rates that are causing Generation Z to have a shorter life expectancy than their predecessors. WTF is going on?

Our model is broken. Any good scientist can tell you that if you keep running an experiment and the results are opposite to what you hypothesized, then obviously your hypothesis is wrong. You need to go back to the drawing board and start again. This is exactly where we're at.

There's a way forward, and I implore you to take action. Read on and apply what you will learn from some of the best experts in the fields of nutrition and health to get yourself sorted out. I learn every day from experts and try to implement and execute new habits daily to ensure I'm at least 1% better than yesterday. I want the same for you, too, because the game we're playing is a long game—the only game in town.

Suicide

Alright, time to get real about a topic that needs addressing.

If you're a man and you're reading this book, odds are you have a buddy or family member who's killed himself. If you're a member of the military or EMS world, those odds go up higher. There were three suicides on my mission, and we were a small deployment of 2000 troops. That's a heavy toll.

The statistics are staggering in the West right now. Men are increasingly killing themselves out of desperation and despair. It breaks my heart when I hear about dads and sons and brave warriors succumbing to the demons that plague their minds.

I'm no stranger to mental illness; I've been dealing with the aftereffects of the war and my inability to right the wrongs that so desperately needed correcting. I struggle to make sense of the senseless. Afghanistan was a fucked up place to be for nearly eight whole months. The culture shock and the death that surrounded it were overwhelming at times. I had a hard time rationalizing what I saw while I was over there, and it affects me to this day.

Our brains are magical machines that scientists have very little grasp of. For instance, what the hell is consciousness? Why am I able to think at all, and why did our brains evolve to allow us to speak, create music, and develop the atom bomb? It's wild, no? I think so. Part of the reason why I love doing what I do with books and podcasts is because I truly believe that humans are here to expand consciousness to the rest of the universe. I think it's a force, like gravity, that is universal, and it will grow at all costs, pulling things towards it with its ever-expanding event horizon.

With that said, our minds can wreak havoc on us as well. Mastery of the mind is something that monks spend their whole lives pursuing, trying to achieve nirvana. It's no wonder, then, that when something traumatizes us, we have a hard time coping with the different components of our brains that handle everything from eating, drinking, and procreating to thought, threat awareness, and social behaviour. The reptilian brain, or the hindbrain, is the ancestral part that makes us behave on instinct. This is what we need to get a grip on, and what Jon Macaskill can help you with in his chapter about mindfulness.

I'm blown away by the statistics for male suicide. There were almost forty thousand male suicides in the U.S. in 2022, with the largest cohort being males between 18 and 44 years old.

This trend is also increasing year over year. These numbers warrant a very close look because this isn't something that appears out of nowhere without cause or aetiology. This must be a symptom of something bigger going on within our societies. But what is it?

With over twenty-two veteran suicides a day in the U.S., how can we possibly keep moving forward with the status quo? Clearly, something needs to be done. Learn more about what is being done by reading both Hal Hughes' and Tom and Jen Satterly's insights.

THE SYSTEM IS FAILING

The signs of stress and inevitable collapse of our healthcare systems are all around us. Diabetes alone is set to completely wreck Canada's healthcare system just through the sheer number of dialysis patients that will need care. It's insane. Not to mention cancer, heart disease, and the nearly 30,000 lives obesity claims every year in this country. Now, imagine if all we needed to do to reverse this was stop putting horrible food in our mouths and go for walks?

As I mentioned earlier, my children's generation is expected to have a lower life expectancy than my generation. That's messed up. Unless there are massive innovations in gene therapy and we can single-handedly reverse disease with some fancy new scientific treatments, these kids are dying due to convenience and a softness that makes it okay to serve them ungodly amounts of sugar but scorn parents for letting them run and bike to the park on their own.

Some sobering statistics:

- In 2020, 1 in 5 children in the U.S. were obese, compared to 1 in 20 in the 1970s.
- 12% of Americans have diabetes, with an estimated cost of $413 billion.
- 1 in 3 Canadians lives with a chronic disease.
- 88% of Americans are metabolically unhealthy.
- Only 5% of North Americans exercise 30 minutes a day.

BE THE CHANGE WE NEED

Learn a thing or two from the ancient scholars, namely the Greeks and Romans. They had their collective act together when it came to being human. Take Socrates' response to one of his pupils.

In his Memorabilia, Xenophon, a student of Socrates, shares a dialogue between Socrates and one of Socrates' disciples named Epigenes. On noticing his companion was in poor condition for a young man, the philosopher admonished him by saying, "You look as if you need exercise, Epigenes." To which the young man replied, "Well, I'm not an athlete, Socrates." Socrates then offered the following response:

"I tell you, because military training is not publicly recognized by the state, you must not make that an excuse for being a whit less careful in attending to it yourself. For you may rest assured that there is no kind of struggle, apart from war, and no undertaking in which you will be worse off by keeping your body in better fettle. For in everything that men do the body is useful; and in all uses of the body, it is of great importance to be in as high a state of physical efficiency as possible.

Why, even in the process of thinking, in which the use of the body seems to be reduced to a minimum, it is a matter of common knowledge that grave mistakes may often be traced to bad health. And because the body is in a bad condition, loss of memory, depression, discontent, and insanity often assail the mind so violently as to drive whatever knowledge it contains clean out of it. But a sound and healthy body is a strong protection to a man, and at least there is no danger then of such a calamity happening to him through physical weakness: on the contrary, it is likely that his sound condition will serve to produce effects the opposite of those that arise from bad condition. And surely a man of sense would submit to anything to obtain the effects that are the opposite of those mentioned in my list.

Besides, it is a disgrace to grow old through sheer carelessness before seeing what manner of man you may become by developing your bodily strength and beauty to their highest limit. But you cannot see that, if you are careless; for it will not come of its own accord."

If you can't see it, let me help you.

By not taking care of your mind, body, and soul, you're being selfish. You're abdicating your responsibility for personal health to the state. Your family and community deserve the best of you, but you refuse to make that happen because it makes you uncomfortable?

Suck it up.

There could be many more pressing issues to deal with right now. If you're reading this, you're already in the top 10% of humanity. So quit your bitching and get to work. Become the savage you know you are.

Reading on in this book, you will find ways to do this. Whether it's from exercise, cold showers, or fasting, these practices prime you to handle hardships and be, as Dr. Jordan Peterson would say, "The person people can rely on at your father's funeral." In the following chapters, you will learn from the best experts on mindset, nutrition, fitness, and recovery. Take notes, do your research, but more importantly, take action.

You can find your own One Week H.A.R.D. Routine at the end of this book to get you started.

Train Hard, Fight Easy.

MINDSET

1

PREPARE YOUR MIND LIKE A SNIPER

Tim Turner & Ben Klick

Getting Up To Speed

I never had the shot at becoming a sniper. No pun intended. It wasn't in the cards for a reservist soldier like myself, and I never thought of myself as a great shot. Plus, the idea of lying prone for days, freezing my butt off, just didn't appeal to me.That said, I am fascinated by snipers. They can bring an entire company of soldiers to a grinding halt. Just one sniper. That's why they're such a valued asset to any commander. If you're familiar with the Battle of Stalingrad or the more recent Bosnian War, sniper warfare was rampant. It paralyzed the conventional movement of forces since any movement outside of their bunker or strong point meant there was a strong possibility that they would get one in the dome from a sniper lurking and stalking his prey. There is a paralyzing psychological effect that snipers exert on their enemies. You don't know where they are, and you don't know when your time is up. It's horrifying, and that's the point. Thankfully, during my time in Afghanistan, I didn't have to deal with any battle-hardened, expert snipers—mostly just poorly trained Taliban who didn't have the marksmanship skills or weaponry to lay down effective fire. But I can only imagine the damage a good sniper team could have done to our morale if they had been stalking us for the better part of our tour. This is why I sat down with Tim and Ben, two of Canada's most distinguished snipers, to talk about the type of person it takes to become a sniper and how snipers must train their minds to be extra resilient in the face of adversity. Their lessons are not just applicable to snipers but to anyone looking to overcome challenges and become a better person. Mental management, as they call it, is your key to success. Here's a bit more from our conversation:

> "Our subconscious mind...moves in the direction of whatever the conscious mind is picturing... If I took a 2x12 and put it on the floor and asked you to walk along it, you'd be able to do that. If I take that same 2x12 and put it forty feet in the air, it becomes a more challenging task... The minute we think about falling, our subconscious mind gets ready to fall... so we focus on the downside, rather than focusing on the task." - Ben Klick

Growth vs Fixed Mindsets

Part of that path included reading and listening. I love to read. I find going into a bookstore exciting. I could spend all day there. Before I had kids, sometimes I did. One book that I got into was *Mindset* by Carol Dweck. She's a Stanford professor and defines people into two categories: those with growth mindsets and those with fixed mindsets. Those with growth mindsets have a "program" in their brain that says, when things get difficult, "I just can't figure this out *yet*." There is the acceptance that one day they will figure it out. It's powerful stuff and a great tool to use with children in a teaching environment.

For those with fixed mindsets, they operate in absolutes: "I either can or can't." We all go through phases of growth vs. fixed mindsets in life. It's normal, but the key is to recognize when you're in a fixed mindset pattern and bring yourself into a growth mindset.

Think back to how your school experience was. Mine was alright, mainly because I had great friends and cool teachers. I was lucky. I realize now that isn't the case for most. I can't say that I was truly inspired leaving high school, but I had some teachers who made teaching look cool enough that I'd want to do it as a career.

I didn't realize school was creating a fixed mindset around my potential. The system is set up to allow parents to go to work and be productive during the day and for the students to one day do the same. It's more cogs in the wheel of society.

Very rigid timeframes, burnt-out teachers, and a top-down curriculum force students into a box where they can't actually move forward on the topics they enjoy the most and have to rigidly hammer away at the topics that provide them the most difficulty. This often leads to remediation and, especially for boys, dropout. Most school systems drastically cut sports and extracurricular activities and eliminated things like shop

DRIVE × GROWTH MINDSET ═ SUCCESS

FIXED MINDSET

$$\frac{\text{GROWTH}}{\text{MINDSET}} = \frac{\text{Belief+Emotional}}{\text{Control+Learning Ability}}$$

$$\text{DRIVE} = \text{Resilience+Aspiration}$$

$$\frac{\text{FIXED}}{\text{MINDSET}} = \frac{\text{Fear+Negative}}{\text{Stories+Doubts}}$$

class and anything outside the traditional academic topics like math, science, and English. All this does is fix the mindset of the student into thinking that all learning is about is the core subjects taught in school, which can really hinder the ability to go out and learn things independently.

Take, for instance, Tim's example from the podcast. His son had a hell of a time understanding trigonometry and only finally got it when it was explained to him in the context of sniping. His mindset shifted from feeling dumb and thinking he'd never get this stuff to a growth mindset where he could confidently apply this math in a high-stress, combat environment. Isn't that something?

> "I was terrible at math in school... Teachers in school don't know how to teach... They don't make it interesting... There's no confirmation until the end... I got math when I joined the infantry... Then, when I went on sniper training, there's a crapload of math... Because this is what I wanted to do, it was easy." - Tim Turner

Ask yourself, what fixed beliefs do you have about yourself that are long established? You're not good at math? You suck at running? You're not a good writer? Most of these probably started when you were a kid and have just never been explored any deeper since you never had the opportunity to try and improve because you didn't believe you could.

You will be exceptional. You just haven't gotten there yet.

My Experience

I can pinpoint exactly when my mindset started to shift. It was sometime in 2017; I was a new dad, working as a high school science teacher, and wasn't in a good place. Things were just not going well. I was hurt, I was depressed, and professionally, I had gone from a pretty cool guy who got to wear body armour and carry a gun to work, to having snotty kids ask me for Kleenex. So, there I was, taking a dump at work and listening to my first-ever episode of the Joe Rogan

Experience podcast. This is relevant because taking a dump at work was one of the highlights of my day. And I'm not joking when I say this, Joe Rogan started talking about how shitty work is for most people and how their highlight is sitting in the toilet, taking a dump, and scrolling through Twitter.

I was like, "Is there a camera in here? How did he know that?"It hit me hard. This clearly shouldn't be all there is in life. Taking a dump and scrolling my Insta feed isn't a good sign that I'm fulfilled. I didn't run out of the school giving my principal the double middle fingers that day, but it put the wheels in motion. Once a new powerful idea takes root in your mind, it's impossible to quell it. It must be brought to a logical conclusion.

Harden Up

This conclusion was that I am not where I'm supposed to be. But where was I supposed to be? That was the start of the journey, the one I'm still on, and the one I'm sharing with you right now.

Practice Your Mindset Improving Self-Talk

Ok, we joked about this in the podcast about Stuart Smalley and how he used to make fun of the motivational speakers from the 80s and early 90s. "I'm special, people like me." It's a great comedy bit from SNL, but as much as we can joke about it, there's a real kernel of truth in using positive self-talk. I use it every day, and it actually works.

Why?

Our brains and bodies are just reflections of our state. If our state is positive and we're convinced that things will go well, our body reflects this and exudes confidence and power. It also works in the opposite direction. Start the day off thinking that it's going to be a rough, shitty day, and your body will manifest that. It may even feel more achy than normal.

Focus on Process, Not Results

Ben made this abundantly clear. You can't do anything to change how others are going to perform; you can't change your targets or the weather, but you can focus on your process. In other words, get super focused on improving your day-to-day habits. Dial them in. Your results will come. Be patient.

"We focused on process, not results... We don't care about results until after." - Ben Klick

Surround Yourself with the People You Want to Be Like

There's a lot of internet lore about a Stanford study that mentioned we're the average of the five closest people in our lives. It's a loose interpretation of the study, but essentially the moral of the story is, winners hang out with winners, and losers hang out with losers. If not, why did your dad forbid you from hanging out with the kids from the sketchy family down the street?

This may seem harsh, but it's reality. You embody the habits and behaviours of the people you surround yourself with. You can apply this to anything that you want to accomplish. Want to become an MMA fighter? Hang out with really good MMA fighters. Want to be a millionaire? Hang out with them. I'm not going to tell you how. That's your job to figure out. I'm sure you can see the other side of this coin now. Hang out with other veterans who still live in the past and blame the VA for all their issues, and you'll never grow and thrive. Get close to whiners and complainers, and you'll become a whiny bitch too.

We are products of our environment as much as our genes. Don't forget that.

Harden up.

2

CHANGE YOUR STORY, CHANGE YOUR MIND

Mark England

Getting Up To Speed

In my conversation with Mark England of Enlifted Coaching, he guided me through a simple exercise: writing out everything that has caused you harm or trauma in the past. He then begins to dissect that story, removing the ugly parts you've clung to for so long that have defined you as the victim. There's a certain comfort in being a victim; it provides a feeling of safety and control. However, in reality, it just erodes your soul over time.Mark provides practical tips on how to identify if you're stuck in a victimhood mentality. The primary indicator, from his experience, is whether you have progressed and grown post-trauma. If the answer is no, then you're likely telling yourself a story that victimizes you and keeps you in the same place.As Mark says,

"There are only two biological states: growth and death."

If you're not growing, you're dying, both physically and emotionally. This has dramatic consequences if you don't heed the advice.

Understanding whether you see events as happening *to* you or *for* you is the ultimate realization. If you believe that an event happened *to* you, then you're likely exhibiting signs of victimhood—thinking "Why me?" or "Life is unfair." On the other hand, if you adopt a stoic perspective and think, "I'm glad this happened *for* me to grow," then life takes on a whole new meaning.

There's never been a better time to be a victim than in this day and age. The internet is screaming for you to be one. You get up in the morning and start getting sucked into a mindless vortex of pity and self-doubt. It's hard not to see the endless spiral of shit most people are heading down, and you can't help but feel a little bad for yourself and your sorry ass too. Right?

Do you think you're immune?

Likely not.

Veterans can be some of the biggest snowflakes when it comes to this mentality. I know because I was one of them and sometimes catch myself falling into this deadly pattern. The scene gets set once you experience a setback, like having a shitty conversation with your wife or you shit the bed on a presentation at work. You slip into the "woe is me" mentality and seek validation for that feeling on your phone.

Hence, the screen sucking.

In the veteran world, this might sound like, "Fuck those civvy pieces of shit. They don't know what we did back in the day for the country. Why can't they respect my sacrifice? How dare they disrespect me?"

Or something like that.

Now that the scene is set, enter stage right with some exogenous substances like booze, weed, or porn, and now you've got a show! The victimhood show, LIVE with Dave.

The question is, why is it so easy to fall into this mindset? Part of me thinks it might be manufactured. With years of data and algorithms, creating pain is a great way for companies to capitalize on it through media. It's an extension of the "if it bleeds, it leads" mantra of the news media, now hyper-focused on you.

> "We're gonna see a bifurcation of people... There are conversations that are weaponized... to further entrench and inflame people's victim mentalities and drive them nuts, then use them as a control mechanism." - Mark England

When you feel like crap, you're more likely to buy useless junk, spend more time online looking for an escape, and disconnect from your reality. It's called "Retail Therapy." Who benefits from your victimhood? Big corporations.

Okay, so fuck those guys, but this doesn't help you get out of the hole, right?

The main reason we fall prey to a victimhood mentality is

the story we tell ourselves. If the story you tell yourself is, "You're a piece of crap, you never deserved this, they did this TO you." You're likely to be in a world of hurt and suffering. This is what victimhood expert Mark England explained in our conversation. Before we delve into what Mark has to say, I want to share how my victimhood mindset has sometimes gotten the better of me.

> "Humanity plus technology plus the victim mentality equals the Borg." - Mark England

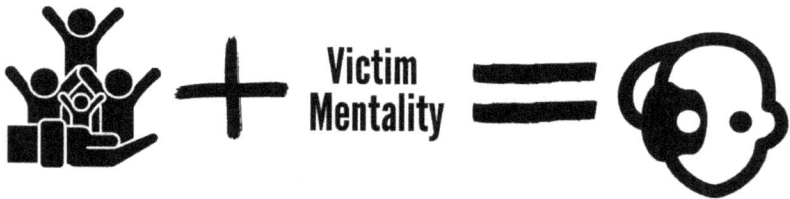

My Experience

I often think, "I should never have gone to Afghanistan." I think that because I see the lack of care from our politicians, military, and civilian population about the war and our sacrifices. It makes me realize that it was all bullshit, and I feel like a fool because I truly believed what we were doing was virtuous and just.

The fall of Kabul in 2021 hit me hard. I was intimately involved with the evacuation of thousands of Afghans who worked with the Canadian government. I desperately needed to get my interpreters and their families out of that hellhole. I committed a lot of my emotional resources to that mission, which did get my two interpreters to safety but left thousands behind.

Through this experience, I realized that our government and military don't care about what veterans have to say about the war. That stung. It still stings to this day. I tell myself they "should" have listened to us. They "should" have been planning for this for years. They "should" have more respect for the sacrifices of their sons and daughters during a decade of war.

All that did was drive me into a deep depression of guilt and rage. I "should" all over myself. The height of the fall of Kabul in 2021 was August 15, the day of my daughter's second birthday party. We had everyone over at the house, and I was in full panic. We didn't have air support or ground support to get our people out, and the Taliban were pouring into the city.

Stories of rape, murder, and mass executions were piling in. I was a complete mess. I couldn't exist in both worlds at the same time. I looked at my family with disgust. How could they be having a birthday party at this time? I had to go for a walk. I cried deep sobs as soon as I was out of sight of my house. This quickly turned into visceral anger without an outlet.

I bottled it up and carried on. I went back inside the house and played the good dad and husband. This wasn't about me today. I wasn't going to ruin my baby girl's day.

But I never truly resolved it. This wound festered, and I wanted nothing more than to burn the whole institution down. The hurt was profound, and I wasn't handling it well. Someone once told me, "Anger is sadness's best friend." This was me in a nutshell—angry, resentful, and keeping a "stoic" face the entire time.

More weed and silent time to take the pain away was a temporary solution, but it wasn't helping in the long term. There was nobody to turn to who "got it." Everyone I had worked with over the last six months was scattered all over the country.

It wasn't until I read a quote that said, "Is your aggressor living in your head rent-free?" that it clicked. Oh shit, the "government" doesn't know me or care about the torment it created. Now I ruminate and feel like they victimized me with the perverse hope that it somehow "shows them" that they're bad people.

Is that really going to do anything? Clearly, the answer was no. I found a lot of peace by latching onto stoic philosophy and began reading Marcus Aurelius' *Meditations* from that point on. It made me realize that catastrophizing and tormenting myself based on a perceived wrong by the government is only causing me harm. For what?

Victim Mentality

I came across this quote from the stoics: "He who angers you, owns you," and it hit me hard. I realized that the government was angering me daily, and now they "owned" me. This was no way to live. My entire world was being affected by this, especially my wife and kids. This was the victimhood cycle that was ruining my life, and I had to break it.

The victim mentality is simply a mindset that allows you to abdicate your responsibility to an external "other" through a story you tell yourself. For instance, my story was, "The government doesn't respect my service or my authority. They should've listened to me and my fellow veterans when we asked for help."Or it could be something like,"I should've never planned that patrol route that got us ambushed where Tim and Bill got killed." Or "She ruined my life and slept with my best friend. She took everything from me!"

These stories get us in trouble because they remove your responsibility from the issues and make you a victim of the event. You now have no control over the situation, and that is very unsettling. The truth is, you always have control over one thing at all times, and that is your mindset and how you perceive even the shittiest of situations.

Viktor Frankl, a Holocaust survivor, makes this abundantly clear in his book, Man's Search for Meaning. Even in the most horrific situations, you can always perceive things however you choose. This is the free will you must tap into to overcome a victim mindset and reframe your story.

Harden Up

Mark has a simple four-step method that can completely reshape your story and has helped severely traumatized veterans and himself. You need to sit with what hurt you and confront it. The process is as follows:

- Step 1: Write it down.

- Step 2: Read it out loud.

- Step 3: Read it at 30% speed.

- Step 4: Read it and pause to breathe after each sentence.

The key is to get your story down on paper. Once you have the whole narrative written down, it can then be analyzed and reshaped to pull you out from being the victim and become the hero.

Harden up.

3

DON'T GET OUTFLANKED

Hal Hughes

Getting Up To Speed

Hal Hughes is a former police officer, MMA fighter, and registered therapist who has faced traumatic brain injuries and addiction. Despite these challenges, he has become a beacon of hope for first responders and military personnel through his therapy clinic.

Hal's career-ending brain injury occurred while he was on the job as a police officer in Ontario, Canada. The injury left him with chronic migraines and an inability to work, eventually leading him to an addiction to opiates. His life took a dark turn.

One remarkable aspect of his recovery is his story of forgiveness.

His assailant was a Native man, and in Canada, there is a restorative justice process aligned with Native customs. Hal participated in this ceremony and forgave the man who had seemingly ruined his life. Hearing how it all unfolded on the podcast definitely caught me in the feels.

In his office, Hal has a bamboo tree, which symbolizes growth and epitomizes his approach to helping others recover from trauma:

"The Chinese bamboo tree is one of these really hard nuts... When you plant it, you've got to plant it in a certain depth of soil, with just the right amount of fertilizer, just the right amount of care, right? Then you've got to water it carefully and give it just the right amount of sun. If you do that every day for a year, nothing happens. Second year... it's down in the dark there in the soil, in the mud, in the dirt... nothing happens. But when it does break through the ground, you can literally sit and watch it grow. And so the question always is: Did it grow that tall in 5 years or 6

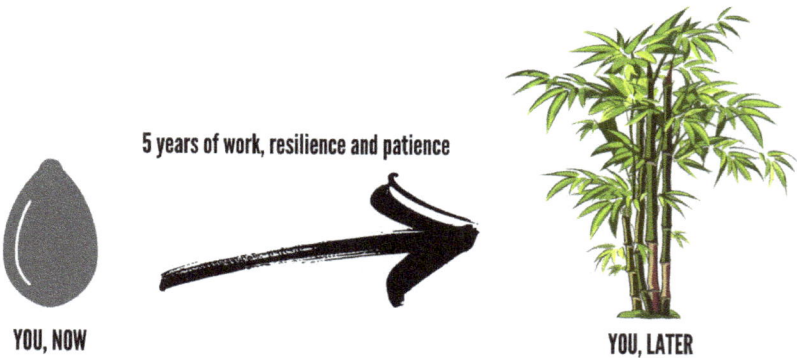

5 years of work, resilience and patience

YOU, NOW

YOU, LATER

weeks? But it had to be in the darkness. It had to be in the soil."

His biggest takeaway is that everyone experiences trauma, and it's of no value to compare yours to anyone else's. We all have different stories and backgrounds; something completely innocuous to one person might be earth-shattering to another.

"Invariably, when you put everyone together in a room and they start talking, the military guys think the cops have it bad because they're working 12-hour shifts, 3 or 4 days a week, not knowing what's gonna happen. Meanwhile, the cops are thinking, man, those military guys—they go overseas, away from their families for 6 months, and they're dropping bombs." — Hal Hughes

At the Veteran Transition Network trauma recovery program I attended, there was a comment about PTSD that stuck with me: "PTSD is about getting outflanked." It's a great analogy. Everyone grows up differently, with unique environments and experiences, so your perception of the world differs from everyone else's. Therefore, one person's traumatic experience in combat may not affect another in the same way.

Your central nervous system is the arbitrator of what becomes held as trauma. There are ways to harden up and be "inoculated" against trauma, but no one is 100% immune. Take my buddy Yves, for example, who shared his experience in Afghanistan on The Hard To Kill Podcast. He had prepared for years to go into combat, mentally readying himself for the worst. Yet, when faced with a situation where he couldn't help a fallen comrade, he felt powerless and outflanked. It's taken him years to recover.

My Experience

My experience wasn't nearly as gruesome, but it affected me nonetheless and caused years of trauma I didn't want to accept. Like Yves, I had always wanted to experience war, fueled by a fascination with GI Joe and the idea of testing myself in combat. I mentally prepared, read extensively on combat and its psychology, and was ready for the possibility of not coming back.

However, my tour was relatively tame—no serious firefights, no explosions. I thought there was no reason for trauma or PTSD, right? Wrong. I had prepared for situations I could somewhat control, like combat scenarios, but I never prepared for the eventuality of building a school and interacting with students.

I had a unique position as a CIMIC (Civilian Military Cooperation) operator, which meant I carried funds to help finance projects in the villages we patrolled to win their hearts and minds. One of these projects was reopening the school attached to our compound. As a teacher, this was an unexpected joy. I helped teach English to the staff and students and learned some Pashto in return. We all worked hard to rebuild that school, and it was fulfilling.

However, two months before the end of my tour, attendance dropped because families were being threatened by the Taliban. The Taliban warned that they would kill the boys if they continued attending school. Some children were indeed harmed. The situation was heart-wrenching.

The worst part for me was seeing a video captured by a local village elder showing kids from the school performing a "bacha bazi" dance for the police chief and village leaders. These events often involve young boys being exploited, and it was beyond disturbing. It went against every moral fiber in my body. Command wouldn't intervene, as it was "their land, their rules." I felt utterly helpless, knowing these atrocities were happening, and I couldn't do anything about it.

I didn't prepare for this. I was outflanked, hard. It's even difficult to write about this because I feel I let those kids down, that I didn't do enough. It hurts to the core. This is where trauma can take root, and why it's essential to recognize that it's not just the hero, knee-deep in combat, who can be hit with PTSD. The key is that PTSD is treatable, and recovery is possible. It's not a life sentence. I've found great comfort in therapy, physical training, and maintaining good lifestyle habits like proper sleep and nutrition. I feel much better now and can run a company, write books, and be a good father.

You'll understand even better after hearing Hal's story that if he can overcome PTSD and get back to helping his brothers and sisters in the first responder world, you can too.

Harden Up

PTSD is a complex issue, so I won't pretend there's a one-size-fits-all solution. However, there are a few things you can do to mitigate its effects and work towards recovery:

Determine if you're suffering from an undiagnosed mTBI and have post-concussion syndrome.

Many modern veterans suffer from mTBIs without knowing it. Multiple undiagnosed concussions can manifest symptoms similar to PTSD. Hal's PTSD was compounded by an mTBI, highlighting the importance of proper diagnosis.

Address poor habits.

Sleep is crucial for good brain and hormone function. Prioritize getting close to eight hours of sleep each night.

Check your hormones.

Many male veterans are unaware that their testosterone levels may be low, contributing to feelings of depression, lack of motivation, and emotional drain.

Seek out a psychotherapist who understands your experiences, like Hal.

The importance of a good therapist cannot be overstated. If you get a bad vibe from one, don't hesitate to switch and find another.

Harden up.

4

MEN ARE DYING FOR A NEW MENTAL HEALTH APPROACH

Dr. Rob Whitley

Getting Up To Speed

Dr. Rob Whitley is a Professor in the Department of Psychiatry at McGill University and a researcher at the Douglas Research Centre. He's also a British military veteran. He strongly asserts that the model currently used to help men recover from mental health injuries is not the one supported by established literature. Let me say that again: the model we use is not the one that the literature supports.

What we typically do now is have men talk it out, face-to-face, with a therapist. This is fine, according to Dr. Whitley, but only for the initial stabilization phase, which may also require medication. However, what shocked me during our conversation was when he said that after stabilization comes the action phase for men. As he says:

> "Start going for walks outside. Go to a market and say hello to a stranger."

Whoa, this isn't what our current model promotes at all. Exercise and being outside? Come on, doc, this sounds like right-wing conspiracy theory.

Dr. Whitley emphasizes that men need to heal "shoulder to shoulder," meaning they need to go out and do something difficult and rewarding in nature with other men, like hunting or wilderness adventure hiking. He even wrote a textbook on the subject called Men's Issues and Men's Mental Health: An Introductory Primer.

But why are men different from women in this regard?

This distinction goes back to our ancestral roles, where men would go out and hunt for the tribe. This was ritualistic and relied heavily on a strong team dynamic. You had to focus on one goal: food. You worked together, shoulder to shoulder, to face your prey. If you were face-to-face, it implied you weren't keeping your eyes on the prize, and your family might starve.

So, you and your buddy would head out, chatting along the trail about how your "cave wife" was nagging you about not opening up about your feelings. Your buddy would listen and provide practical advice or not. But at the end of the day, you hashed out what was bothering you and felt a massive sense of accomplishment when you brought home dinner.

Have you ever noticed that men tend to open up in the car while driving or on the couch watching TV? It's not weird;

it's just hardwired into us to avoid deep conversations while looking into someone's eyes. This isn't crazy; it's just science.

Or have you noticed that baby boys tend to look away more than baby girls? Boys, in general, often avert their eyes from their mom when being talked to, which can sometimes frustrate mothers. This behavior is influenced by testosterone levels in the fetus and could explain social behavior differences in adulthood.

Women, on the other hand, lived among themselves in the community and would chat face-to-face. They need that eye-to-eye contact to feel connected in the conversation. My belief is that since the therapy world is predominantly female, talk therapy face-to-face has become the norm, which is devastating to men's mental health outcomes.

Let's Talk

If you're Canadian, you've likely seen or heard of the Bell Canada "Let's Talk" initiative to end the stigma around mental health. I think it's a huge steaming turd of bullshit.

Let me explain.

This corporate initiative aims to promote mental health awareness. But what is "mental health awareness"? The goal is to make it easier for people to ask for help when they're suffering. Ok, great. But what does it do to address the underlying problem?

Does it help address the crippling soullessness of Western society? The devastating effects of loneliness on men? It's the second leading cause of death for men under 50, and 75% of all suicides in Canada are by men.

Sure, let's get talking, but then what? Like the push-up challenges and all the other bullshit initiatives out there, do 30 push-ups and all your troubles and your buddy's troubles disappear with each pump of your arms?

I can't help but see this as lazy. It's everywhere, especially in Canada. We pay lip service to everything but take very little practical action to fix things. Words, not deeds, the complete opposite of what our elite JTF-2 special operations unit would say. We love to enact new laws and legislate away our problems. Let's give veterans free weed, let's have safe injection sites for everyone, let's not keep violent offenders behind bars and let them out on bail.

Some of these ideas may come from a place of compassion, but the reality is, most just make things worse if the underlying root issue isn't addressed. This takes work and lots of quantifiable, empirical evidence, which is exactly what Dr. Robert Whitley has provided.

I'm going to get straight into it: the cult around mental health isn't doing us any favors. The morning talk show hosts propagate the myth that we just need to talk it out more. The military doctors separate a soldier from his team to "work on his mental health." The parents let their kids screen-suck all day and then pay thousands to see a therapist who gladly takes their money. These are all the cultists that bow down to the god of talk therapy.

This approach isn't working.

Have You Seen the Veteran Suicide Numbers?

Over 30,177 American veterans have committed suicide since 9/11.

Suicide rates are four times greater than combat deaths.

COVID lockdowns increased suicides by 16% within the American military.

The rate of suicide among male veterans was 3.8 times higher than that of female veterans.

Younger male veterans (under age 55) had a significantly higher risk of death by suicide than other male Canadians. This was greatest in veterans under age 25, where the risk was 2.5 times higher than other male Canadians of the same age.

Veteran Suicide Deaths, 2001-2021

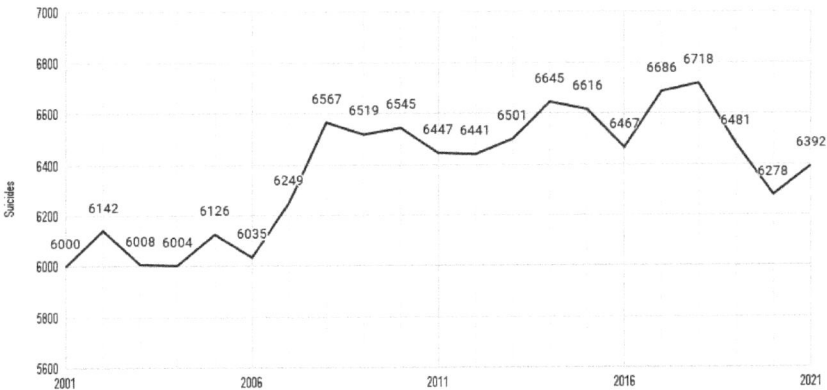

Data based on a slide from Veterans Affairs (U.S.) annual report on veteran suicides (Courtesy of VA)

My Experience

I have never been truly suicidal, but I have felt like I should just hide away from society. I have a good idea why things spiraled out of control for me. I was a new dad, recently released from the military, working a new job that I didn't find fulfilling, gaining weight, in substantial chronic pain, and lacked a deep connection with my wife or anyone else. I was simply existing from day to day. It really got dark some days.

But you know what changed it all for me? Action.

I took control of my life by getting a coach and training religiously every week. I joined a competitive sports league. I started hunting and fishing with my in-laws. These seemed like random decisions, but Dr. Whitley's research shows that what I did is exactly what men, especially veteran men, need to do to heal from mental health injuries.

Harden Up

Dr. Whitley's thesis is simple: get outside and do challenging things with your friends. Hunting, fishing, hiking, canoeing—you get the point. This might be easier said than done. Our lives can present roadblocks to taking action, like having no friends in your area or swearing off being in the wild since leaving the Army.

Here's a list of amazing veteran-friendly organizations and activities you should definitely check out. Don't wait to take action. Go out today and walk in the park or down Main Street. There are benefits to just being active around people, even if they're civilians.

Warrior Adventures Canada - This program brings CAF veterans and RCMP members together on a multi-day wilderness adventure to help heal from a career of service. (https://warrioradventures.ca/)

Irreverent Warriors - For veterans only, this group organizes "Silkie Hikes" where you walk around in your "silkies" all over the U.S. and Europe. (https://irreverentwarriors.com/)

Operation Flow State - A BJJ and psychedelics retreat in Mexico for veterans and first responders, where you learn how to fight and open up about your biggest issues. (https://www.becomingom.com/vets)

Voluntold - This app turns your walking and workout data into a game where you can compete against other veterans. You can create local communities of veterans to go walking with. (www.voluntold.co)

Harden up.

5

ADDICTION CAN RUIN YOU

Dr. Robb Kelly

Getting Up To Speed

Dr. Robb Kelly is a fascinating individual. I first came across him via email, and as I read his bio on LinkedIn, I thought, "Wow, this guy is on fire!" He's been featured on mainstream media and talk shows, and he's the author of Daddy Daddy, Please Stop Drinking. His work in California has helped many people overcome their alcohol addictions. What struck me as unique in his approach was his focus on the "addictive brain" as the main paradigm keeping people, including himself, addicted to alcohol for so long. This was a new concept for me, so I delved deeper.

The "addictive brain," as Dr. Kelly describes it, is a brain that has a need. In his case, this need was alcohol. His need for alcohol led him to violently attack his wife and nearly destroy his entire life.

Dr. Robb Kelly didn't just stumble into success. He fought his way through significant struggles, including battling alcoholism from the age of nine. His first drink was on stage before a musical performance. For Robb, it was like,

"The whole world had changed."

Robb went on to become an accomplished musician, playing with Queen and Elton John, and earning £1000 an hour, which helped him pay for Oxford med school. According to Robb, alcoholism is not merely a volume problem. The Mayo Clinic states that for men, consuming more than four drinks a day or more than fourteen drinks per week puts you at risk for alcoholism. However, Robb believes it's a combination of two factors:

- Being born with an addictive brain.

- Experiencing childhood trauma.

According to Robb, self-sabotaging neural pathways define the addictive brain. The hypothalamus controls our primal urges, but for alcoholics, instead of receiving normal signals to eat and drink water, it tells them to drink alcohol.

"All signals are being sent to have a drink."

Parenting can also influence the addictive brain in some children. Not feeling worthy is a driving force, so treating your kids poorly can increase the expression of the addictive brain.

In one of Robb's accounts of an alcoholic binge, he describes his overwhelming need to drink, putting aside professional and family obligations. But when he went to grab a drink of vodka, he had a remarkable revelation: instead of drinking straight from the bottle, he grabbed a crystal glass. Why?

"Alcoholics drink from the bottle."

Alcoholism acts differently from other addictions. Robb believes that alcoholism is something you're born with. While other drugs require consumption in volume to become addictive, alcohol can hook you from your first drink, making you think, "Wow."

My Experience

Based on Robb's definition and my experience, I can safely say that I don't identify as an alcoholic. However, I do have what might be considered quasi-addictive habits, like mindlessly checking my phone at night and feeling anxious about missing important messages.

In my younger years, particularly in the 90s and early 2000s, I would drink heavily on weekends. It was just part of hanging out, getting drunk with friends, and having fun. I never craved alcohol but enjoyed the social aspect. According to the government, however, I would have been classified as a binge drinker, which is a red flag for potential alcoholism. But does that mean all my friends were alcoholics too? We used to joke about this, and fortunately, none of us ended up grappling with full-blown alcoholism.

This reminds me of a Jim Jeffries skit about Queen Elizabeth II. He jokes that if you have 14 drinks a week, you're considered fine, but if the Queen has four cocktails a day, "She's a full-blown alcoholic." He then humorously describes her chasing

Prince Philip around the house.

I bring this up because it's important to discuss the concept of high-functioning alcoholism. Like Dr. Kelly, some people can maintain a seemingly normal life while being crippled by their addictions at home. This is common among those who serve. I've seen Sergeant Majors so intoxicated at 2 am that I figured they'd never make it to PT at 0500, only to see them there as if nothing happened, ready to do it all over again the next night.

In Canada, alcoholism affects 4.2% of the population, or about 1.3 million people. This rate has increased recently due to events like global lockdowns and the general feeling that the world is going to hell. There was an 18% increase in alcohol-related deaths from 2019 to 2020, the largest year-over-year change in the last 20 years.

Harden Up

According to Dr. Kelly, the first step is acknowledging your problem and seeking help. Help can come in many forms, but his method begins with identifying why the problem exists and then following his multi-step program.

The truth is, 70% of people struggling with alcoholism will relapse, but that rate declines the longer someone stays sober. Dr. Kelly emphasizes the importance of finding the help you need to recover. He even offers his own number for those who are hurting to reach out.

One of his most significant insights is the "7.3 seconds" rule. From his research, he discovered that an alcoholic has 7.3 seconds to shift from self-harm to self-care and stop themselves from drinking. This is where Robb's method has its greatest impact.

His insights are many, but he's spot-on when he states:

> "Alcoholism is the only self-diagnosed disease in the world."

As he explains, no test can prove you're an alcoholic; only you can have that self-realization. Dr. Robb Kelly's approach focuses on addressing the root cause of alcoholism, targeting the disease itself rather than just the symptoms. He highlighted the impact of childhood trauma on neural pathways and self-destructive behaviours, emphasizing the need to rewire habitual thinking. This approach is explained in the chapter, Change Your Story, Change Your Mind with Mark England.

Harden up.

6

BE MINDFUL LIKE A NAVY SEAL

Jon Macaskill

Getting Up To Speed

Mindfulness is a topic I often delve into because it allows me to examine how I think and feel about things. But what's the difference between mindfulness and meditation? Good question.

Jon Macaskill, a retired Navy SEAL commander, was a team member of the infamous Operation Red Wings, where all but one "lone survivor," Marcus Luttrell, were wiped out in Afghanistan. Jon discovered mindfulness and meditation because he couldn't continue "living the dash." Living the dash, as he describes it, refers to living from the date of birth to the date of death on your tombstone as "the dash"—a period with nothing of great importance, marked by numbness. He felt emotionally numb and was also numbed by the medication he was taking.

"I couldn't live the dash anymore." — Jon Macaskill

He realized he needed to change. He began with a simple mindfulness practice that I think everyone should incorporate into their daily routine. It goes something like this:

Take a two-minute pause during your day to sit, close your eyes, and take a few deep breaths. Just focus on your breathing and your feelings. It's normal to have random thoughts or get distracted. When you're done, open your eyes and carry on with your day.

There's a lot of research on meditation and mindfulness. The science community often refers to it as transcendental meditation, but we'll stick with "meditation" for simplicity. It has been shown to have a significant effect on stress levels and the primary stress hormone, cortisol. Chronic stress is a major contributor to disease and inflammation, with over 75% of Americans experiencing high levels of stress.

Studies have also shown that meditation can increase your lifespan by significantly reducing the chances of burnout from stress. For example, healthcare workers who performed two 20-minute meditation sessions per day for three months saw significant improvements in outcomes such as insomnia, anxiety, and burnout.

A massive, often overlooked benefit is that meditation can train you to be more present with your loved ones. In my case, it helps me be more present with my kids. We're so distracted

MEDITATION GUIDE

SCAN ME

by phones and work that we rarely get the chance to just be in the moment.

For veterans, evidence is emerging that mindfulness training can reduce suicide rates. Improving problem-solving skills and dealing with stressful situations seems to reduce the instances of suicidal thoughts.

My Experience

For me, meditation is more "formal," and I use it as a way to start and end my days (sometimes). I use a breathing technique called The Wim Hof Method, which we'll discuss in a later chapter with guest Brandon Powell (Breathe Mother Fucker). I find meditation particularly beneficial because it leaves me feeling relaxed and calm. But meditative practices can occur during other common activities too. For example, a morning run you do at the same pace with the same route can be meditative if it helps clear your mind.

By definition, meditation involves focusing or clearing your mind using a combination of mental and physical techniques, while mindfulness is the awareness of one's internal states and surroundings. They're very similar. I view mindfulness as something I can practice without having to stop, close my eyes, and rest with my thoughts. For instance, if I'm getting upset during a conversation with my wife about who has unloaded the dishwasher more often, I become mindful of why I'm getting upset and try to mitigate that emotion. Then, I become mindful of any sarcastic comments I might make. See how it works?

Harden Up

If you spent any time in the Canadian Army during the Global War on Terror, you likely learned how to box breathe. It's a simple breathing technique to get your prefrontal cortex back online when you're stressed out and one of my preferred methods for meditation.

There are numerous breathing techniques, of which I'm only beginning to understand, and I encourage you to research them further. Refer to the chapter "Breathe Mother F*cker" for more.

Breathe In

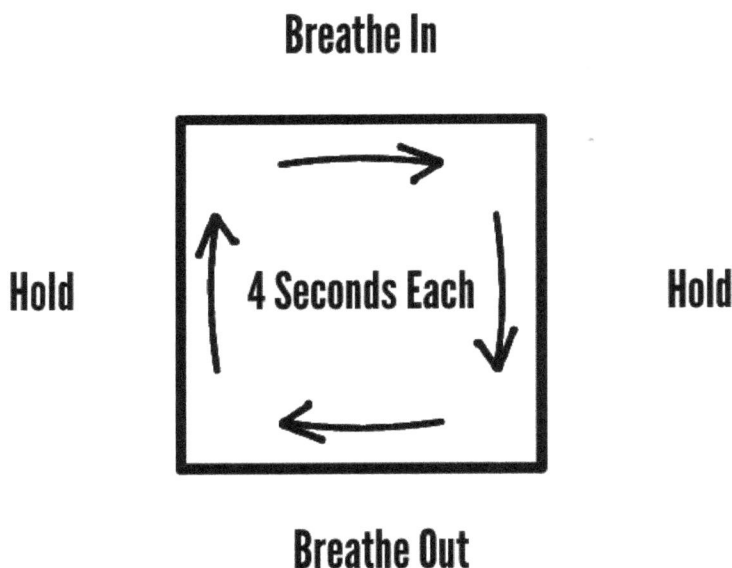

Hold — 4 Seconds Each — Hold

Breathe Out

Box breathing is simple: breathe in for four seconds, hold for four seconds, breathe out for four seconds, and then hold for four seconds. When my kids are driving me nuts and I'm starting to lose it, I revert to box breathing. We used it in combat in Afghanistan, and sometimes it feels like I'm under fire at home. I've taught my kids to breathe when they get stressed out too. They know when I'm box breathing that I'm trying to calm down, and sometimes they calm down as well, though often they don't, so I have to intervene—but I can do it more calmly, rather than like a recently divorced warrant officer with a drinking problem.

Back to Jon.

Having Jon Macaskill on the show was a real treat. He's forging ahead with his podcast, "Men Talking Mindfulness," and his mindfulness coaching business, "Mindful Frogman." When you realize that even the most elite warfighters on the planet deal with the same issues as the rest of us, it puts things into perspective. We're all human and have to deal with the challenges of life.

Harden up.

THE LIONS ARE HOME FROM WAR

Stuart Scheller

Getting Up To Speed

When it comes to standing up for what you believe in, few can match Stuart Scheller. A retired Marine Corps Lieutenant Colonel, Stu publicly criticized the US military's general staff following the disastrous retreat from Afghanistan in 2021, which left 13 American soldiers dead.

In uniform, Stu bravely posted a video online highlighting the failures of command. Then the fallout began. His book, *Crisis of Command*, is a compelling read and embodies the true definition of courage in the modern era.

Stu is a true warrior, having fought in the Global War on Terror for over a decade. He believed deeply in the mission. He was what we'd call a "troop favorite" because of his leadership style—he understood the fight and literally got in the trenches with his men. But as he recounts in his book, things started to shift during a mission in Afghanistan that left him questioning the purpose of their fight.

He was receiving briefings from troops on sentry posts around the camp, all saying the same thing: "We keep getting attacked from Pakistan, just over the border, and we can't do anything about it."

To Stu, it seemed mind-numbingly stupid not to pursue the Taliban into Pakistan. But politics prevented it. Fast forward to 2021, and the U.S. had done nothing to prepare for a withdrawal from Afghanistan. Interpreters, embassy staff, and billions of dollars worth of equipment were to be left behind, with the Taliban expected to take over.

As chaos unfolded, I played a significant role in the Canadian effort to save our interpreters. The level of unmitigated failure shocked me and caused deep emotional pain. As the Taliban marched into Kabul unopposed, I went on national television to express my disbelief and utter disappointment with the Canadian government. But I wasn't in the military anymore; Stuart was.

The circus that surrounded Stuart was surreal. He was ridiculed, jailed, humiliated, and revered. The US military didn't know how to handle him. Meanwhile, his family life was falling apart. His wife had warned him not to do anything that could jeopardize his career for the sake of the family. But Stuart felt that holding the US military and government accountable was more important than his personal life.

His wife followed through on her warning and filed for divorce, taking their three boys with her. As Stuart said during our conversation:

> "The metric for me being a good father isn't the amount of time I spend in my suburban home with them but the principles I'm willing to stick to and uphold."

That stuck with me. Today, a father's worth seems tied to his time spent at home rather than the principles he stands for and the values he instills in his children. This is something I want to convey to my children as well—there must be a line in the sand. If you don't stand for something, you'll fall for anything.

My Experience

Real talk: The COVID-19 "Pandemic" was a totalitarian dream come true. Every wannabe dictator came out to play, whether at the mall, church, on Twitter, or in government. For the weakest-willed, this was their Super Bowl. Men who couldn't lift a barbell over their heads if their lives depended on it were telling people like me that I was the problem and would kill their grandma for not wearing a mask or getting vaccinated. Gyms had to be closed to the healthiest people on Earth because, #trustthescience.

Shame can erode your principles, let me tell you. It works even better on people without principles. I don't have many principles, but here they are:

Be kind to myself and others.

My body is my vessel to do good; treat it well.

Never make a bad situation worse.

I could refine those points, but that's probably for another book.

During the COVID era, I didn't stick to my principles. I'll be honest, I didn't do well during that period. My entire worldview was collapsing. I believed that our government, despite its incompetence, still had our best interests at heart. That belief eroded daily.

Looking back, I realize it was because I couldn't reconcile the idea that if I chose not to receive a medical treatment, that choice wouldn't be respected. In the Canada I grew up in, we valued individualism. That was what was sold to me, anyway. During the pandemic, politicians suggested putting the unvaccinated in "camps" and labeled them as racist and misogynist, part of a "fringe minority."

I lost trust in every institution.

The shame I felt after receiving my second shot was profound. My wife, mother, family, and the media all shamed me into getting a medical procedure I didn't want. What stung the most was that they knew I had a valid point. They knew I wasn't speaking irrationally and had never made wild, unsupported claims. I graduated from one of the best universities on the planet with a science degree. I wasn't an idiot or a political zealot.

The reason I bring this up is that as soon as I took that shot, I felt misaligned. I hadn't adhered to one of my principles. The person I was in public didn't match the person I was in private. This is why Stu Scheller's story is so compelling—he is exactly who he says he is, both in public and private. This was never more apparent than during the fall of Kabul in 2021.

Stuart has been called every name in the book, lost his family and career, and been thrown in the brig, yet he has always maintained that there needs to be accountability for military failures at the highest level. He's a principled man, and his book *Crisis of Command* is a testament to that.

Having been in Afghanistan for eight months, I couldn't agree more with his reasoning. I genuinely thought I was going there to win a war. However, it became apparent that there was never a vision of winning—only "pushing the ball down the field," as Stuart explained it. Generals were content to create PowerPoint slides about how many bad guys they killed or how many projects they completed, only to hand it off to the next guy a year later.

I liked Stuart's criteria for waging war: A four-star general should get the job of winning the war and commit to ten years of fighting. If not, step aside for someone else, and if no one is willing, maybe we shouldn't be fighting the war.

So, when 13 American troops are killed in front of the Kabul airport, and the withdrawal from Afghanistan is a disaster, someone should take responsibility and allow for accountability. This is what I expect from leadership.

I think Stu summed it up well regarding the connection between military leadership's accountability and soldier suicides:

> "I can only imagine how many suicides would be prevented if leaders just accepted responsibility."

Harden Up

One of the last lines in Stuart's book, *Crisis of Command*, is:

> "The lions are home from war. And we're not assimilating."

The biggest takeaway from speaking with leaders like Stuart is the concept of "post-traumatic growth." This message resonates with me because I've had my issues with the war, but it also allowed me to grow emotionally, physically, and professionally. I knew war would be challenging and reshape me. I'm grateful for my war experience and cherish the privilege of having lived like a lion on the battlefield.

I hope you're living like a lion.

Harden up.

FITNESS & NUTRITION

8

EAT LIKE YOUR ANCESTORS

Ben Azadi

Getting Up To Speed

As the saying goes, "We are what we eat." This couldn't be more evident in our modern era. There's both a metaphorical and literal aspect to this expression. Literally, our cells are made up of what we consume. This is a fundamental reason why many of us are sick, dying, and miserable. And I'm not alone in thinking this way.

Ben Azadi is on a mission to help 2 million people break free from the "Standard American Diet" (SAD) and lose weight through the keto diet. The keto diet is the polar opposite of SAD, emphasizing a much higher intake of fats—70% of calories from fat, 20% from protein, and 10% from carbohydrates—compared to SAD's 60% from carbs, 30% from protein, and

10% from fat. The difference is stark: one diet is carb-heavy, and the other is fat-heavy. Which one do you think is healthier?

"We're stuck as sugar burners... We're never accessing the body fat, and that's gonna lead to a lot of problems... and it's gonna make you easy to kill." — Ben Azadi

You don't need to consult scientific papers or doctors to see the difference. Just look around. Try finding a lean person in a crowd at a mall or water park—it's challenging. Even the perception of being lean has shifted to people with higher than 15% body fat. Seeing someone at 20% body fat might make you think, "Wow, that guy is looking pretty ripped." That's how far our standards have shifted towards fat and out of shape.

Ben discussed his journey towards keto on the podcast and how he's helped thousands of people unlock what he calls ancient healing.

Our current diet was engineered by politicians—the same ones who told us there were weapons of mass destruction in Iraq and assured us things were safe and effective. In the 70s, the American food guide emerged, marking the first time politicians decided what people should eat (even the English didn't dictate what the Irish should eat during the famine).

If you're old enough to remember the children's show *He-Man* and *Transformers* on TV, you know what I'm talking about with the "Food Pyramid." Looking back, it was pure propaganda, plastered all over houses, schools, and doctor's offices, and it was total, industry-driven nonsense.

The Industry-Designed Food Pyramid of Death

The base of the pyramid was whole grains, followed by

vegetables, fruits, meat, and fats at the top. This setup implied that we should eat more from the bottom than the top. And like good little soldiers, we followed orders, stuffing ourselves with processed, grain-based foods. Breakfast became "the most important meal of the day," and cereal sales soared. I loved my massive bowl of Frosted Flakes every morning, with skim milk, of course. I didn't want the fat in my milk to make me fat. Then I'd polish that off with a big glass of orange juice. The 80s were amazing.

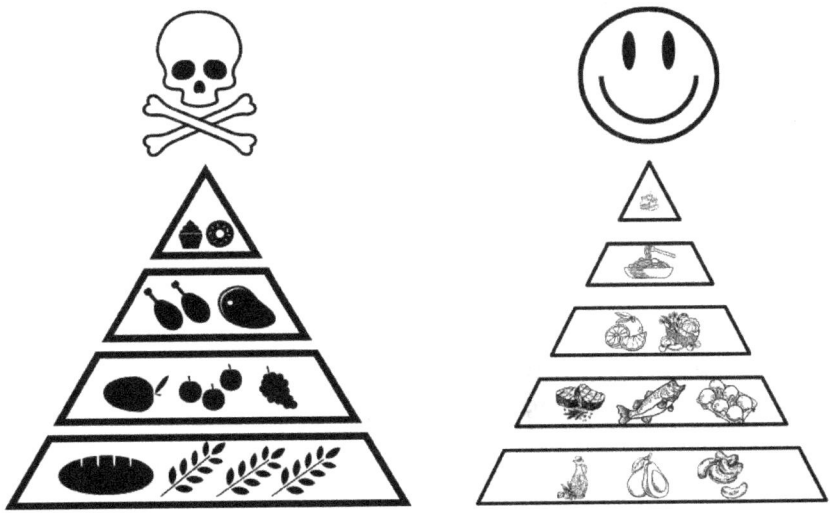

Compare that to how we traditionally ate: primarily meat and animal fats, with a few seasonal fruits and vegetables. Breads and rice were present but not in the convenient, sliced forms we see today. Refined sugar only became widely available during the Victorian era and was a luxury for the rich and royal. I got the following quote from a New York Times article from 1986:

"Victoria enthusiastically endorsed 'tea time': it promoted products of the British Empire. As this daily interlude expanded into an elaborate ritual, so did the royal girth. Her subjects, dutifully imitating their monarch, likewise took to the proliferation of sweets with similar results."

If sugar were the only culprit in our toxic food environment, the battle might be easier. But in the 20th century, industrialists found a way to profit from industrial seed oils. Originally used to lubricate machinery, these oils were repurposed for human consumption, replacing lard and butter. This led to the rise of canola, grapeseed, and vegetable oils—cheap and effective at preventing food spoilage, but harmful to our health, causing inflammation and other issues.

But Isn't Fat Good for Us Now?

Yes, it is. Fat won't kill you, but the source of your fat is crucial. Ben Azadi advocates for a high-fat diet, commonly known as the keto diet, which involves your body entering ketosis. He argues that our bodies function much better in this state.

"[We're] sick and tired of being sick and tired."

Ketosis is a metabolic state where the body uses fat reserves for energy instead of carbohydrates. This requires minimal carbohydrate availability in the bloodstream and low glycogen levels in the muscles and liver. If these reserves are full and you consume more carbs, the excess is stored as fat. Our bodies are highly efficient at storing energy.

Fat is essential for survival, providing energy when food is scarce. It's stored around our bellies, close to our center of mass, to avoid hindering movement. In ketosis, your body consistently accesses fat stores for energy, leading to various benefits like less brain fog, reduced sleep needs, and more consistent energy levels.

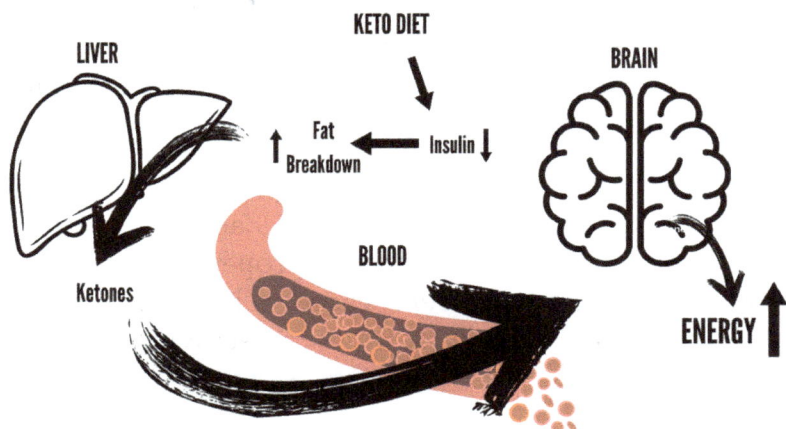

My Experience

I spent nearly a year on the ketogenic diet in preparation for an Ironman competition, completing the event while in ketosis—a fact I'm proud of. After researching and calculating, I realized that consuming the required amount of carbohydrates during the race was impractical for someone my size. Instead, I went keto: six months without beer or cakes, but plenty of macadamia nuts and coconut milk. I completed the Ironman and felt fantastic.

In ketosis, your body uses ketones rather than glucose to produce ATP, the energy molecule. Ketones are more efficient, producing 50 ATP molecules per long-chain fatty acid, compared to 30-32 ATP per glucose molecule. This results in better energy production and overall well-being.

"There are no essential carbohydrates." — Ben Azadi

Ben combines the ketogenic diet—a 70% fat, 20% protein, and 10% carb ratio—with fasting. We'll delve deeper into fasting in Cynthia Thurlow's chapter (Fasting for Longevity). The main concept is that combining periods of not eating with a low-carb diet maximizes your body's fat-burning potential, eliminating the need for "diets."

However, the transition to keto isn't simple. My first attempt at "going keto" was a disaster. I tried to eat loads of fat, primarily cream cheese and olive oil, without proper planning. I was miserable and, after two weeks, caved in by ordering a large fry and Coke at McDonald's. It was a carb-craving meltdown.

Harden Up

As Ben explains, this is a process. First, you need to wean yourself off the "crack" of sugar. Then, you can adjust your macros and ensure you track your food intake. Prepare your kitchen with the necessary foods to succeed, not just cream cheese.

Start with a detailed meal plan for the week. The principles are simple: eat meat, eggs, and non-seed-derived oils and fats. My favorite meal is steak and eggs with a bowl of high-fat yogurt and blueberries.

Here's a recipe for "fat bombs" I created to fuel myself during the Ironman without resorting to sugary gels:

Harden up.

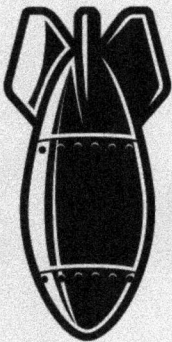

FAT BOMBS

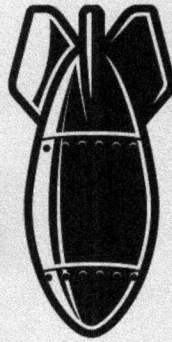

- 1 can of high-fat, all-natural coconut milk
- ½ cup of cream
- 1 cup of frozen blueberries
- 1 scoop of LeanFit whey protein powder
- ½ tsp sea salt

Blend and pour into an ice cube tray, then freeze.

9

FASTING FOR LONGEVITY

Cynthia Thurlow

Getting Up To Speed

Fasting is all the rage right now; it's like the latest cool thing everyone's trying. But what exactly is fasting? Technically, it's going without food for at least 24 hours. Anything less is just skipping a meal. This distinction is important because certain cellular processes kick in only after a full day without eating, providing numerous health benefits.

I had the pleasure of chatting with Cynthia Thurlow, a renowned expert and author of *Intermittent Fasting Transformation*, about the benefits of fasting for health and longevity. Research from the University of North Carolina at Chapel Hill reveals that 88% of Americans are metabolically compromised, suffering from obesity, high triglycerides, insulin resistance, or high blood pressure. Fasting can be a powerful tool to help reverse these trends.

Fasting isn't new; humans have been doing it since the dawn of our species. We're built for long-range hunting and enduring periods without food. Unlike other animals, we're not the fastest or the strongest, but we excel at walking, running, and hunting over long distances, even without food. A common myth is that we'll be low on energy if we don't eat regularly, but that couldn't be further from the truth.

> "I think in our modern-day lifestyles, when we're conditioned to believe that snacks and mini meals are the way to maintain our health, I'll be the first person to say that that couldn't be farther from the truth." — Cynthia Thurlow

If we became weaker and less energetic as soon as we stopped eating, we wouldn't have survived as a species. What actually happens is that our body starts using stored energy reserves. First, it taps into blood glucose, then glycogen stored in the liver and muscles, and finally, it accesses fat stores. This process is essential for burning off the fat we've accumulated over time.

Fasting is a way to activate this natural fat-burning mechanism. One of the key benefits, as Cynthia explains, is a process called autophagy. This process helps remove cellular waste, reducing inflammation and promoting healthy cell regeneration. Another major benefit is improving insulin resistance.

> "Your body goes in and takes out the trash." — Cynthia Thurlow

Insulin Resistance

Insulin resistance is a crucial issue that more people should be aware of. Insulin is the hormone that regulates blood sugar levels. If your blood sugar is too high or too low, it can be life-threatening. Diabetes is a condition where insulin production or function is impaired, meaning sugar passes through the blood without being absorbed.

In the past, doctors would test for diabetes by tasting a patient's urine for sweetness—if it was sweet, you had diabetes.

So, what is insulin resistance? Imagine you have highly skilled soldiers fighting off terrorists in your neighborhood. If the terrorists keep coming, the soldiers eventually wear out and you need more, less effective soldiers, to go to battle. This is what happens with insulin resistance: your body's cells become less responsive to insulin, leading to chronic high blood sugar levels even though you're producing more and more insulin.

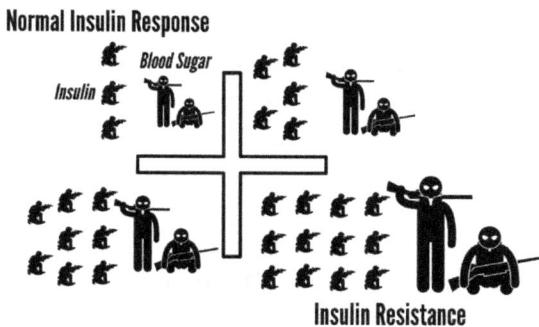

This condition can eventually lead to diabetes if not managed. Fasting gives your "soldiers" or insulin a break, allowing your body to recalibrate and better manage blood glucose. This is why Cynthia advocates incorporating fasting into your routine. According to the American Diabetes Association, diabetes costs the U.S. $412.9 billion, with over 10% of the population affected.

Stress Control

Cynthia emphasizes that fasting isn't for everyone, especially if you're stressed. Stress causes the body to release cortisol, a hormone that increases blood glucose levels to prepare you for a "fight or flight" response. Chronic stress leads to constant cortisol production, which can cause burnout and weight gain.

Fasting adds another layer of stress, known as eustress, which can be beneficial in moderation. However, if you're already stressed, adding fasting to the mix might not be a good idea. It's important to assess your stress levels, whether through a smartwatch or by tuning into your body's signals.

For women, Cynthia advises against fasting during menstruation, pregnancy, or illness.

My Experience

I started fasting in 2017. Initially, skipping breakfast was daunting. I was a firm believer in "breakfast is the most important meal of the day," thanks to years of eating sugary cereals. The first morning without breakfast, I felt a mix of

SAMPLE SCHEDULE:

- **Mon/Tues**: Intermittent fasting (no breakfast)
- **Wed**: Normal eating
- **Thurs/Fri**: Intermittent fasting (no breakfast)
- **Sat**: 24-hour fast
- **Sun**: Normal eating

fear and hunger around 9 AM, tempted to stop for fast food. But I resisted, and the hunger passed.

Afterward, I experimented with longer fasts—24 hours, then 48, and eventually 72 hours. You can watch my 72-hour fast journey in the Veterans Getting Fit AF community. I lost nearly 10 lbs and gained control over my eating habits, eliminating the fear of low energy.

Harden Up

Here's a simple fasting protocol I use with my athletes in the B.E.A.S.T. program, borrowing heavily from Cynthia and Ben Azadi (Eat Like Your Ancestors). The big caveat is that you need a solid nutritional foundation first:

- Eat at least 1g/lb of your desired body weight in protein daily.

- Eliminate junk food and sugary snacks.

- Hydrate and eat like an adult, not a child.

- Incorporate healthy fats like butter and coconut oil without worrying about cholesterol.

Step 1: Skip breakfast and see how you feel. (You still need to consume the same daily calorie intake as if you had three meals.)

Step 2: Skip breakfast two days in a row, then eat normally for one day. Repeat this cycle. Skipping breakfast isn't a full fast but helps you adjust to not eating and manage hunger.

Step 3: Continue the above routine but add a full 24-hour fast once a week. This is where you'll see significant benefits, including fat loss.

INTERMITTENT FASTING 101
(Your Quick Start Infographic)

TYPES:
The 3 most basic types are:
- 16:8 - Fast for 16 hours and eat during an 8 hour window almost every day.
- Warrior Diet - Fast for 20 hours and overeat for 4 hours during a 24 hour period.
- Eat-Stop-Eat: Eat as you normally would all week and incorporate one or two 24 hour fasts.

BENEFITS
- Improved insulin sensitivity
- Decreased body fat
- Improved autophagy
- Better hunger awareness
- Improved growth hormone synthesis

HOW IT WORKS
IF acts by improving insulin sensitivity since the pancreas, which secretes insulin, is given a rest. It seems that the increased rest periods between eating windows helps increase nutrient absorption and decreases the window in which glucose can be stored as glycogen which can eventually be converted into body fat.

HAZARDS
If you are under an unusual amount of stress such as injury, psychological distress, pregnant or experiencing any major shifts in your life - avoid IF for now. Fasting was forgiven by our forefathers in our religious texts and you should do the same. IF imposes a good stress on the body but throwing that on top of too much bad stress will compound your problems.

This straightforward approach removes the guesswork. Combined with daily walking, especially while fasting, you'll see significant improvements over a few months.

Fasting is a powerful tool for health and longevity. However, it's crucial not to overdo it, especially with longer fasts over 48 hours. In North America, and particularly among veterans, there's a tendency to believe that more is always better—more money, more success, more fasting. That's not the case. Balance is key.

In many religious traditions, fasting is practiced once or twice a year to purge the body and activate autophagy. I typically do two 72-hour fasts annually, with a few 24-hour fasts in between. There are no hard rules; it depends on your metabolism and body. The main thing is to have a solid nutritional foundation before you reap the full benefits of fasting.

How to Break Your Fast

When breaking your fast, prioritize protein and either carbs or fats, but not all three together or just carbs and fats. This approach helps manage insulin sensitivity, which spikes after a fast. Cynthia recommends high-protein Greek yogurt with blueberries and a touch of natural honey. I prefer a cup of homemade bone broth. Have this light meal an hour or two before a larger meal, ensuring you're not overly insulin-sensitive when you eat.

Fasting is a tool that, when used correctly, can be a game-changer for your health.

Harden up.

10

CHOLESTEROL WON'T KILL YOU. POOR METABOLIC HEALTH WILL

Dr. Philip Ovadia

Getting Up To Speed

Talking with Dr. Philip Ovadia a few years ago was one of the most transformative conversations I've ever had. It significantly improved my life and made a profound impact on the Hard To Kill Community.

Dr. Ovadia is a cardiac surgeon and author of *Stay Off My Operating Table*. His mission is to debunk the "Diet-Heart Hypothesis," which has contributed to the rise in obesity, diabetes, and coronary heart disease over the past 50 years. You may not have heard of this hypothesis, but it's the reason grocery stores are filled with "low-fat" products like crackers, cereal, and foods loaded with high fructose corn syrup. The hypothesis, rooted in Ancel Keys' biased and flawed study, unfairly demonized fat and cholesterol as the primary causes of coronary heart disease (CHD).

My bold claim for this chapter: Ancel Keys is responsible for more deaths than any other person in history. His industry-funded research led people to drastically reduce their intake of saturated fats and animal proteins, while metabolic diseases skyrocketed.

Dr. Ovadia draws a line in the sand, stating that enough is enough. He realized that both low and high cholesterol patients were ending up on his operating table. This revelation led him to question the validity of the high cholesterol = heart disease narrative. He had a wake-up call and lost over 100 pounds by rejecting the advice that had led him to become severely obese and metabolically unhealthy.

The Diet-Heart Hypothesis

The Diet-Heart Hypothesis suggests that consuming more saturated fats, which contain cholesterol, leads to higher blood cholesterol levels. This idea is overly simplistic and flawed. Cholesterol is vital for life, with 80% of it produced by our bodies and only 20% coming from our diet. Thus, eating fatty meats isn't the primary cause of elevated blood cholesterol.

Dr. Ovadia likens the misconception about cholesterol to blaming firefighters for fires simply because they are always present at the scene. Cholesterol is present in the arteries of individuals with cardiovascular disease because it's part of the body's repair process, not the cause of the disease. The real culprit is the damage caused by excessive sugar consumption, which leads to small scars in the blood vessels. Cholesterol arrives to patch these scars, but if the damage is extensive, it leads to atherosclerosis, narrowing the arteries and potentially causing heart attacks.

The solution, according to Dr. Ovadia, isn't to reduce cholesterol or rely on statins. Instead, it's about changing your diet to eliminate sugar and incorporate healthy fats and proteins. Dr. Ovadia now helps thousands of people escape the misleading diet-heart hypothesis and reclaim their health.

Absolute vs. Relative Risk Reduction From Statin Use

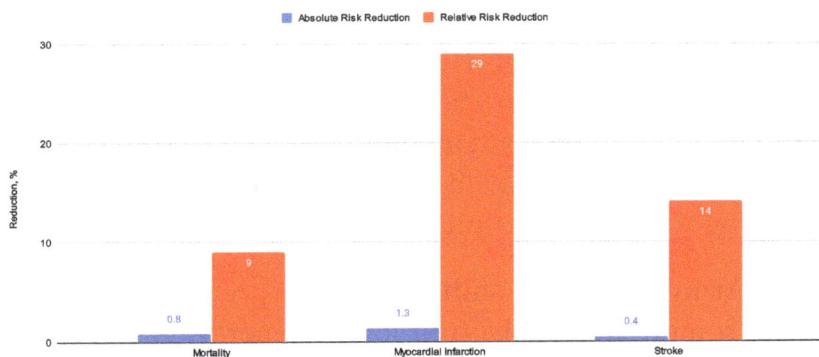

Source: Evaluating the Association Between Low-Density Lipoprotein Cholesterol Reduction and Relative and Absolute Effects of Statin Treatment, JAMA Intern Med, 2022

My Experience

Growing up, I was always known as "Big Dave." I was a large kid, and before puberty, I was chubby. Compared to today's standards, I might have been leaner, but at the time, I wasn't at an optimal weight. This affected my self-confidence but also motivated me to embrace fitness. My dad was my original fitness role model. He used to run up Mount Royal in Montreal and return drenched in sweat, sporting short Adidas shorts and a headband. When I was about seven, he started taking me to the community gym, teaching me how to use the machines and dumbbells for some classic

Schwarzenegger-era workouts.

Being chubby made me self-conscious, especially at the pool, where I refused to take off my shirt, claiming I was fair-skinned due to my Irish heritage. In reality, I had developed gynecomastia, a condition typical in chubby boys going through puberty or men using anabolic steroids. I struggled to find a solution, resorting to push-ups and ghetto bench press setups at home, but nothing worked. I also played football, hockey, and swam, but my "chub" persisted.

At 14, after reading Men's Health, I decided to cut all fat from my diet, believing it was the solution to my weight issues. I eliminated butter and salt, ate more tuna and skim milk, and indulged in low-fat foods like Frosted Flakes and crackers. I was living the low-fat dream.

In the Army, my views shifted slightly. I realized that I was always somewhat chubby and low on energy. A PE teacher once told me that eating fat in the morning kept him going better than carbs like oatmeal and bread. Following his advice, I started eating margarine sandwiches in the field, and surprisingly, felt great. My body responded well to the extra fat, even if it wasn't the healthiest kind.

As I got older and wiser, I revisited the idea that perhaps eating more fat could help control my weight.

Harden Up

If this is your first encounter with the concept of metabolic syndrome, good. It's arguably the single most important concept to grasp for becoming "hard to kill." Dr. Ovadia defines metabolic syndrome as having any one of the following five issues:

- Obesity
- High blood triglycerides
- Insulin resistance
- High blood pressure
- Low HDL cholesterol

A staggering 88% of North Americans would fail this test and be considered metabolically unhealthy. This condition is the primary cause of pain and suffering in our society, but it's reversible, and not with the help of Big Pharma.

According to Dr. Ovadia, you can completely reverse these metabolic issues by following these simple steps:

- Don't smoke.
- Don't drink.
- Exercise for 20 minutes every day.
- Don't eat sugar or processed foods.
- Eat adequate amounts of protein daily.
- Consume healthy fats daily.

It's not complicated but requires a paradigm shift. Imagine the savings in medical bills, lost wages, and long-term health costs if you did these five simple things every day instead of relying on doctors and Big Pharma to make you "healthy."

Harden up.

11

BRAZILIAN JIU-JITSU:
MORE THAN JUST CHOKING PEOPLE TO DEATH

Dr. Gino Collura

Getting Up To Speed

You know how to tell if someone practices BJJ? They won't stop talking about it.

Brazilian Jiu-Jitsu (BJJ) has become a significant trend, especially among veterans, but it has also exploded globally over the last decade. Thanks to the rise of MMA and the influx of veterans from the War on Terror, there's a growing interest in this martial art.

Dr. Gino Collura, a PhD who has conducted research on the positive effects of BJJ on veterans' psychology, is a prime example. He's a badass, having worked extensively in law enforcement both at home and abroad, including in Colombia. He has a keen understanding of what it takes for veterans to become "whole" again, and he sees BJJ as a crucial piece of that puzzle.

According to Dr. Collura, many veterans gravitate towards BJJ because it provides a controlled environment for expressing combativeness. Veterans, having been trained to kill, have a unique need for an outlet for their aggressive instincts. While this capacity for violence exists in all humans, the military refines it to a sharp edge.

> "For veterans, the warrior ethos doesn't just disappear once they leave the military. Jiu-Jitsu provides a way to reintroduce that ethos and continue building their identity in a meaningful way." — Dr. Gino Collura

Dr. Collura's research suggests that the intimate, face-to-face combat in BJJ allows the central nervous system to calm the mind, especially for those with PTSD. It enables the body and mind to engage in the "fight" mode of the fight, flight, freeze response, which can be beneficial.

Why?

PTSD often results in an inability to turn off the fight, flight, freeze response. Engaging in physically demanding activities helps redirect the mind away from unwanted thoughts. Exhausting the body through combat sports like BJJ can help veterans regain control over these responses.

Dr. Collura explains that many veterans develop a deep distrust of others due to their experiences in combat, where anyone not in uniform could be a potential threat. This distrust can lead to a persistent state of hypervigilance, exacerbating PTSD symptoms. BJJ helps rebuild trust by adhering to a strict code: when a practitioner taps, signaling submission, the match ends. This code of honor, if broken, can result in expulsion from the gym, which resonates with veterans' ingrained sense of honor.

> "Practicing Jiu-Jitsu offers a chance to reset your brain, providing a reprieve from worry and stress. It acts as a form of mental conditioning, crucial for emotional regulation and well-being." — Dr. Gino Collura

BJJ challenges participants to face their fears, an element often lost in today's comfort-driven culture. By engaging in this physically demanding and potentially dangerous activity, practitioners confront their primal instincts and grow stronger.

My Experience

Brazilian Jiu-Jitsu, or BJJ, originated in Japan and was brought to Brazil by Mitsuyo Maeda, a Japanese judoka. Carlos Gracie, a Brazilian, learned the art from Maeda and taught it to his sons, who then spread it worldwide. The Gracie family's prominence in events like Pride Fighting and the UFC helped popularize BJJ.

I was first introduced to some basic BJJ techniques in the military, such as arm bars and dealing with heavy opponents. I later embraced the sport with my son, diving deeper into the BJJ community. The camaraderie and shared experience remind me of *Fight Club*: once people know you're "in the club," they seek you out.

Before classes, I often feel a mix of dread and anticipation. It's not fear of injury or mistreatment but rather a confrontation with my "inner bitch," as Joe Rogan puts it—the part of me that wants to stay safe and avoid discomfort. However, after each class, I feel alive, accomplished, and ready to protect my family if needed. BJJ also aligns with Dr. Whitley's research on how men recover from trauma through action rather than discussion, reinforcing a sense of belonging and purpose.

Harden Up

Being part of the BJJ community introduces you to some fantastic people. One such person is "Blitz" TJ Kreutzer from the We Defy Foundation, which funds a year of BJJ training for veterans. This initiative is an excellent way for American and Canadian veterans to start their BJJ journey in a veteran-friendly gym environment.

Dave Szwoboda has also created a unique retreat in Mexico (becomingom.com) that combines BJJ with plant medicine, helping veterans and first responders process deep-seated trauma. These retreats address not only the emotional aspects of trauma but also the physical and metaphysical, filling a gap left by traditional approaches.

Harden up.

12

THE HARD TRUTH ABOUT ERECTILE DYSFUNCTION

Dr. Judson Brandeis & Dr. Elliot Justin

Getting Up To Speed

Let's have a real conversation about a sensitive topic: your penis.

Ladies, this chapter is for you too, as you likely have a man in your life who could benefit from this information—and you'll enjoy the benefits of a healthier penis as well.

Here's the deal: 40% of men in their 40s experience erectile dysfunction (ED), and this percentage increases by 10% with each subsequent decade. ED can be defined as the inability to maintain an erection during sex, difficulty achieving an erection, or erections that are not firm enough—what doctors sometimes refer to as "pushing rope."

I dedicated a whole chapter to this because it's crucial for your overall health. I spoke with two incredible doctors to understand how big of an issue ED is, particularly among veterans.

First, I chatted with Dr. Judson Brandeis, a urologist with extensive experience working with veterans. He revealed that the VA is one of the largest buyers and suppliers of Viagra and Cialis globally, indicating a high prevalence of ED among veterans. One significant factor is PTSD, as medications like SSRIs, often prescribed for PTSD, are notorious "cock killers." While ED medications can provide a temporary fix, they may mask more serious underlying health issues.

Big picture: ED can be an early warning sign of cardiovascular disease. Dr. Brandeis explains that the small blood vessels in the penis are more prone to blockages, which can also indicate similar issues in the heart's larger vessels. If left untreated, ED can precede a coronary event.

Another expert, Dr. Elliot Justin, pointed out that doctors rarely inquire about their patients' sex lives or the sexual side effects of medications. This oversight can leave significant health issues unaddressed.

> "The data that we're generating is going to become the standard of care for evaluation of sexual health. My goal is to have sexual health become not something that a doctor asks as an afterthought if you maybe have a problem because you're a vet. But ask everyone, because someone's sexual health is key to their self-esteem and overall health." — Dr. Elliot Justin

According to Dr. Brandeis, men should typically have 4-5 erections per night as a form of "exercise" for the penis. Without regular nocturnal erections, the penis may start to shrink. This could be a sign of low testosterone, a critical factor in maintaining sexual function. If you're not waking up with morning wood, you might have low testosterone, especially relevant for veterans exposed to endocrine-disrupting pollutants.

My Experience

The decline in testosterone levels among men in the Western world is alarming. Factors contributing to this include poor diet, lack of exercise, exposure to xenoestrogens, and sleep deprivation. For veterans, toxic exposures during service may play a significant role. The average healthy testosterone range is 400 ng/dl to 1200 ng/dl, but levels have been dropping over the past 50 years. This decline is inversely correlated with rising obesity rates.

Mean Total Testosterone Change in Men

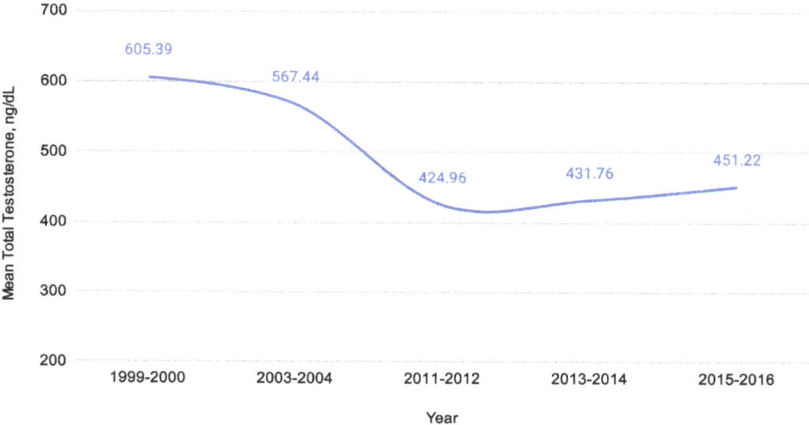

I discovered that my testosterone levels were below 400 ng/dl despite lifting weights, eating clean, and sleeping well. This revelation led me to consult with my doctor about potential causes, including toxic exposures during military service. While my sexual health remains good, the issue of low testosterone is ongoing and requires attention.

I created my BE.A.S.T. Body Blueprint Program to help men improve their testosterone levels through lifestyle changes before resorting to testosterone replacement therapy. This program is available to members of my Veterans Getting Fit AF community.

Dr. Brandeis also emphasized that maintaining healthy testosterone levels can protect against heart disease, enhancing both sexual function and cardiovascular health—a win-win.

In our conversation, Dr. Brandeis mentioned Dr. Elliott Justin's invention, the FirmTech Ring®, a device that monitors nocturnal erections and sends data to your phone via Bluetooth. This "DickBit" provides objective data on penis health, similar to how an ECG monitors heart health.

> "If my number of nocturnal erections went down, I have a vascular problem until proven otherwise. So it's actually a better indicator than blood pressure or an electrocardiogram because minor variations of those don't tell you much of anything." — Dr. Elliot Justin

Tracking nocturnal erections can provide an early warning system for cardiovascular issues, allowing for lifestyle changes before serious medical intervention is needed. Your penis could literally save your life.

Harden Up

Dr. Brandeis offers similar advice to Dr. Ovadia (see: Cholesterol Won't Kill You Poor Metabolic Health Will):

- Stop smoking.
- Exercise daily for at least 20 minutes.
- Avoid alcohol.
- Eat adequate protein and avoid junk food.

Following these guidelines can resolve many ED issues, provided they aren't psychological. Other negative effects of ED include depression and strained intimate relationships. Many men dismiss their sexual health, viewing it as unimportant or shameful. Unlike other health issues, sexual dysfunction remains a taboo topic, even with doctors.

As an infantry grunt, I wouldn't leave you without a scientifically proven way to increase the size of your hammer. This isn't a gimmick; it's based on the "P-Long Study" conducted by Dr. Brandeis, which has undergone peer review. The study outlines a protocol for penis enlargement, including medications and a penis pump, which you can find in the linked peer-reviewed paper.

If this chapter is the only thing you take away from this book, I'm happy. But don't keep this knowledge to yourself; share it with a friend or buy them a copy. However, be cautious: one participant in the P-Long Study reported that his wife couldn't handle his newfound girth.

Harden up.

(literally)

13

DESTROY DAD BOD

Jason Khalipa

Getting Up To Speed

Chatting with CrossFit Games champ Jason Khalipa was a big deal for me. I got into CrossFit in 2008 after my platoon challenged me to do Fran. It crushed my soul, and I realized there's a whole other level of fitness that I had no idea about. Jason is also a BJJ champ, author of *As Many Reps As Possible*, business owner, and father. His 2008 CrossFit Games win was one for the ages when the sport was just starting to take off.

Jason is passionate about being a role model for his children. His social media feed showcases this, as he often shares moments of grappling with his son and daughter, ensuring they can handle themselves physically. He's a BJJ champion, if you were wondering. This is just what elite performers do.

Regarding "dad bod," the pop culture term for the physique of a middle-aged man who has a softer, pudgier appearance, Jason believes it's a travesty to accept being out of shape. He views being overweight and unhealthy as a decision and has taken on the responsibility of changing the paradigm. Jason envisions "dad bod" as being characterized by 15% or less body fat, presenting a physical specimen that children can look up to.

"The dad bod should be a physically fit, strong male. That should be the standard." — Jason Khalipa

The reality is that 44% of veterans are overweight or obese, which is five percent higher than the national American average. Recent research has shown that overweight dads significantly increase the risk of their kids developing type II diabetes and obesity. These conditions are precursors to metabolic disease, the leading cause of death in Americans and Canadians.

I wholeheartedly agree with Jason. If I'm willing to die for my kids, you know I'm damn well ready to be healthy for them. And you should be too.

My Experience

In 2008, I was a platoon second in command. The troops posted daily workouts on the team whiteboard. When I saw the rep count for "Fran" (21-15-9 reps of pull-ups and thrusters at 95 lbs), I remember asking my troop who challenged me if it was a joke. He said, "No, Sarge. That's the workout." About thirty minutes of torture later, I spent the rest of the week consuming copious amounts of Advil and laying in bed when

I wasn't on duty.

I was hooked, though.

Something about the masochistic side of me took over. I had been looking for something this hard for years but couldn't find it. Needless to say, I went down the rabbit hole. I started watching the games on YouTube, fanboying my favorite athletes, with Jason being one of them. I used the CrossFit system to get fit for my deployment to Afghanistan, and it kept me moving and dialed in during those 50-degree days, wearing 80 lbs of gear and humping over grape fields for six hours.

I learned tons from the community, too. The *CrossFit Journal* was awesome. I discovered legends in the strength and conditioning game like Bill Starr and Mark Rippetoe. I began changing my paradigm around nutrition by hearing lectures from Gary Taubes and learning about folks like Dr. Kirk Parsley (see *Sleep or Die*) and Mike Bledsoe of the *Barbell Shrugged* podcast. My horizons broadened, and I became more aware of how much I didn't know. It was very humbling.

Fast forward to the present day, and I'm literally talking about fitness and health with Jason Khalipa. Our conversation focused on how to design fitness and health goals around longevity and practicality.

Harden Up

Jason discussed the baseline standards all men should maintain throughout their lives, no questions asked:

100-yard sprint: Jason points to a troubling viral clip

of a mother sprinting away from an out-of-control tractor trailer with her baby. Another equally terrifying video shows a mother losing control of her baby in a stroller that rolled toward oncoming traffic. She couldn't catch up because she was obese and unfit, but fortunately, another man intervened at the last second. Don't let that be you.

Bodyweight deadlift: You should be able to lift someone your size off the ground. Full stop. Not being able to do so may mean you can't carry your wife or children out of danger. The deadlift is a foundational movement that needs to be part of everyone's longevity plan.

Get off the ground: You should be able to get up off the ground quickly and without support. No mention if groaning due to years of ruck marches is permissible, but I think Jason would give us a pass as long as we meet the standard.

"If you're a grandma, if you're a grandpa out there, do you think that your kids are gonna want you to watch their kids if you can't lift them up? Hell no."— Jason Khalipa

The Proficiency Pyramid

Jason has a great way to conceptualize how he sets up his training, which I call the Khalipa Proficiency Pyramid.

At the base is fitness. No questions asked. Use the standards above to determine what you should focus on, or refer to the conclusion of this book and use my workout guide. Once fitness is covered, the next focus should be skills. Skills like first aid are crucial since they are most likely to be used. After first aid, Jason focuses on combatives, and finally, firearms training.

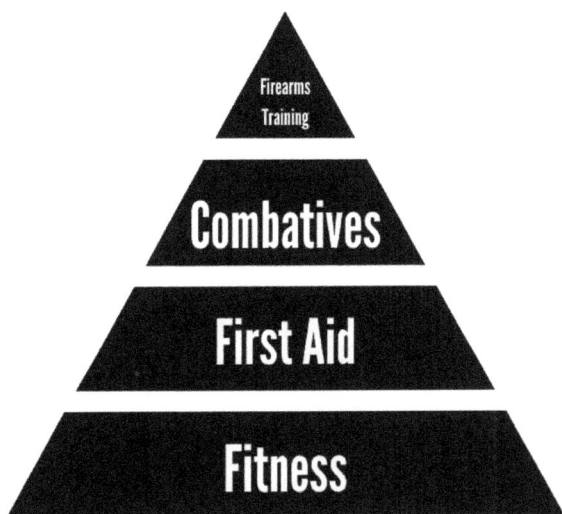

I don't know how Jason never ended up in the military, but I'm glad he's on our side because he's a stone-cold assassin. His reasoning for improving skills is based on a hard-to-kill philosophy. He believes in protecting himself and, more importantly, his family from danger.

Protect Your Kids

On a final note, Jason emphasizes the importance of exposing children to challenging experiences early on to develop healthy, strong, and resilient individuals. He trains his kids in grappling and firearms, teaching them to handle themselves. He rightly points out that bullies are often weak, insecure people who project their insecurities onto others. The best way to guard against bullying is to develop children who are strong, confident, and capable. If more kids spent time on the jiu-jitsu mats and less time on video games, we might see a very different world in 20 years.

"It's a great thing,especially in the social media day and age, to expose your children to hard things because life will get hard. They will face adversity. And it should be our job as parents to expose them to adversity in a very effective, safe manner." — Jason Khalipa

Harden up.

RECOVERY

14

SLEEP OR DIE

Dr. Kirk Parsley

Getting Up To Speed

I first heard Dr. Parsley on a friend's podcast before podcasts were even cool. The conversation blew me away, and I immediately Googled him. I started reading his blog posts and doing some extra research for my own professional development.

Being a Navy SEAL is cool, but being a doctor who addresses sleep issues that SEALs have is even cooler. Kirk's perspective is unique because he's experienced the week-long exercises of no sleep, being pushed to the limit and beyond. You don't have to be a military veteran to experience massive amounts of sleep debt either. As Kirk explains, most Americans are sleep-deprived. It's an epidemic.

We have devalued sleep over the last half century, and we're seeing the repercussions: premature death, accidents, poor grades, and medicating our kids for misdiagnosed ADHD. The list goes on.

Let's dive into what sleep research is telling us.

About one hundred million Americans are sleep deprived. The economic impact of poor sleep is staggering. Research reports that the US economy can lose up to $411 billion annually due to insufficient sleep.

Dr. Parsley isn't joking when he says that not sleeping will kill you. Approximately 32% of Canadians aren't getting enough sleep. According to a massive meta-analysis of sleep data, mortality nearly doubles when people get less than seven hours of sleep per night.

The study found, "[those] who had cut their sleeping from seven hours to five hours or less faced a 1.7-fold increased risk in mortality from all causes, and twice the increased risk of death from a cardiovascular problem in particular."

So, approximately thirteen million Canadians aren't getting enough sleep and are going to die a bit earlier – SO WHAT?

I've got Netflix and Call of Duty to play!

The effects of poor sleep are widely studied, and Dr. Parsley lays them out clearly. Having worked with the SEALs allowed him to identify a few key performance indicators that can be solved with better sleep. According to Dr. Parsley, the world's most elite warriors came to him with all sorts of issues, including:

- Brain fog
- Fat gain
- Increased injury rate
- Poor emotional and impulse control

Kirk summarizes it succinctly as: "FATTER, COLDER, DUMBER, SLOWER"

Operator Syndrome

Dr. Parsley observed that many Navy SEALs were suffering from performance issues rather than physical injuries. This led him to identify a pattern he called "Operator Syndrome." He found that low anabolic markers, high estrogen levels, high inflammation, and poor insulin sensitivity were common among these individuals, urging him to investigate the impact of sleep on their performance.

One surprising finding was the prevalent use of the sleep aid Ambien among special forces soldiers. Dr. Parsley discovered that Ambien not only interfered with the quality of sleep but also reduced essential deep and REM sleep. Deep sleep is known as the most anabolic time for physical recovery and muscle growth, while REM sleep is critical for cognitive processes such as memory consolidation and emotional processing. Dr. Parsley emphasizes that Ambien, especially when combined with alcohol, further exacerbates these negative effects.

> "I took Ambien almost every night...it destroys about 40% to 60% of the quality of your sleep. So it's a net negative. You're losing sleep by taking sleep drugs."—Dr. Kirk Parsley

Dr. Parsley's research demonstrated the transformative effects of improving sleep on soldiers' performance, mood, cognition, memory, motivation, and overall health. By discontinuing the use of sleep drugs and alcohol, these individuals experienced remarkable improvements in various aspects of their lives. He also discussed chronic insomnia, highlighting its detrimental impact on life expectancy.

> "Chronic insomnia is associated with a lower life expectancy of about ten to twelve years. Chronic use of sleep drugs is the same. I don't think the sleep drugs are doing anything to cause death. I think it might be accelerating the decay because you're lowering the quality of your sleep." – Dr. Parsley

My Experience

What Kirk was saying about sleep really struck a nerve with me. As an infantry guy, I had done loads of training that left me super worn out and with the superpower of being able to fall asleep anytime, anywhere, at a moment's notice. Add a tour to that, where sleep was often interrupted and spotty for eight months, and I knew something wasn't optimal about my sleep and recovery.

I lost my mind a few times, sitting in a hole I dug, trying to stay awake on day three of a defensive training exercise. Staying up for seventy-two hours isn't good for your brain. I would see bears and people that weren't there. I remember one exercise where a guy couldn't take it anymore and just ran into the woods screaming. Being able to push through fatigue is definitely an acquired skill. I remember pulling all-nighters in university, mainly because I procrastinated until the last minute. Or the sleepless nights when my kids were newborns, then hopping in a car and going to work to teach all day. I don't think I could've done it without the years of practice in the infantry.

My main concern these days is the damaging effects of chronic sleep deprivation on my testosterone levels. Study after study shows massive dips in testosterone levels for Army Rangers on exercise and troops returning from deployment. The research isn't promising. If you thought you could just take a two-week vacation on the beach and nap away the years of deployments and Ripit nights, you're wrong. The damage may be permanent. At least I have a superpower to be able to sleep anywhere at any time.

Harden Up

Sleep hygiene is super important, and Kirk asks, what would your ancestors have done one hundred thousand years ago? Here are some simple habits to implement:

- Put down your phone, nerd (at least one hour before bedtime)
- Black out your bedroom (no blinking lights or TV)
- Cool down your room to Paleolithic cave temperatures (17 degrees Celsius)

According to Kirk, if you do this, your sleep quality should improve dramatically. However, don't be fooled by its simplicity; this is surprisingly hard. I guarantee you'll come up with all sorts of excuses not to do one of these. I know I do!

Kirk says: "If you need to watch that one more episode on Netflix, go to bed, set your alarm one hour early and watch it...no one is gonna do that."

Harden up.

15

CONTROL YOUR PAIN AND STAY SUPPLE

Dr. Kelly Starrett

Getting Up To Speed

I have to be honest: I'm a total fanboy of Dr. Kelly Starrett. Since I got injured, I have watched probably every one of his MWODs on YouTube, subscribed to his mailing list, own all his books, and even did a CrossFit Open WOD at his box in San Francisco. He was also the inspiration for my book, *The Nimble Warrior*. So, getting him on my podcast early on was a total thrill. Kelly is the author of *Becoming A Supple Leopard, Deskbound, Ready To Run*, and *Built To Move*.

It was a total shot in the dark, but I've always believed in the concept I learned in the Army: "don't ask, don't get." So, instead of believing that a newbie podcaster couldn't land a NYT bestselling author, I said, "fuck it," and sent him an email.

Thanks to my podcast padawan, Andy from The Rugby Coaches Corner podcast, for introducing me to Kelly. We linked up, and you can now behold all the awesomeness we covered in just an hour.

There's so much more to cover here, but the gist is simple: We Can Do Better.

When it comes to training our warfighters, we need more people like Kelly saying, "Hey, you can be doing this a lot better and for cheaper." If we had that, guys like me might still be serving.

As I discussed training with KStar on my podcast, we dove into the concept of mobility. If this is your first time hearing about mobility in training...where have you been? It's probably the single most important modality that has been missing from all our training plans. I'm sure you do flexibility exercises and, like everyone I train, say that your flexibility is shit. I get it; mine isn't great either. The more important question to ask yourself is, how's your mobility?

The difference between flexibility and mobility can best be described by this analogy: Imagine you have an elastic band and you tie a knot in it. If you stretch that band, it still gets longer, but you've still got a knot that keeps everything tighter than it has to be. It lacks full range of motion. This is what mobility training seeks to fix. Sure, you might be able to touch your toes, but can you pop a deep squat or push your hips back to adopt a great deadlift position? This is where mobility training really helps create a more well-rounded athlete.

Kelly's favorite saying is, "Practice makes permanent." So make sure what you're "practicing" won't lead you into years of pain and misery. This concept is relevant when applying it to mobility and injury prevention training. As I learned, you won't improve your back pain if you only do two marathon mobility days a week. You have to do a little bit every day.

One great point Kelly made about our warfighters is this: When we have a tank, it's a serious piece of equipment worth millions of dollars. We take care of it, maintain it, and make sure not to lose or destroy it prematurely. However, this concept doesn't apply to the most important resource of any military: its manpower. Imagine if each soldier were deemed an asset and not just a "plug" or "grunt," and they were all seen as performance athletes. We would then ensure that their health and performance were maintained at the highest levels. Although this may seem like a massive added cost, as Kelly puts it:

> "How many soldiers are you losing every year to preventable musculoskeletal injuries? And if we can bring that down by ten percent, that would pay for itself in the reduction in recruiting and training costs."

My Experience

Once I started following Kelly's Mobility WOD after I got injured, I began to understand why I got injured and how to start fixing my issues. They were all mobility and strength issues developed over years of practicing the same shit over and over again, poorly.

Like most folks in the Army, our physical training consisted of running, more running, ruck marching, push-ups, and pull-ups. We never touched a barbell or did any flexibility or mobility work, unless you count the grizzly French Canadian warrant officer telling us to bounce when touching our toes before a run in his purple running tights.

I thought I was fit as fuck. By Army standards, I was. However, I was super weak. Thinking back, I would've shit my pants if I had to pull two hundred and twenty-five pounds off the ground. This fundamental lack of strength and poor mobility eventually led to my back injury. Not realizing how bad my injury was didn't help either. I didn't do anything to make it better until I was forced to. So, instead of feeling sorry for myself, I started doing exercises that Kelly recommended in his book, *The Supple Leopard*.

Harden Up

Starting a mobility program is crucial to your long-term survival. There's an old man who lives down my street, and he's so bent over to the side that he ties his dog to the other side to counterbalance him. He's me in twenty-five years if I don't keep working on my mobility, and you're likely in the same boat too.

At right is a simple protocol that I started with to improve my squat. The squat is one of the most fundamental movements, and doing it well requires good mobility in all joints.

If you'd like more on how to recover and prevent injuries, download my Injury Prevention Guide.

Get at it and...

Harden up.

SQUAT IMPROVEMENT PROTOCOL

Squat Test: The most important part – cold test of 10 reps (pay attention to any tight areas in your ankles/calves/hips). FILM YOURSELF FROM THE SIDE and watch later.

Single Leg Glute Bridge: Ten reps/leg (pay attention to tight areas around hip and low back)

Banded Good Morning: 30 reps

Poor Man's Hamstring Curl: 30 reps total

5 Way Hips: 3 full sets per leg

Banded Hip Distraction: Minimum 1 min/side or until your hips feel more open

TFL SMR: Hold on tender spots for 30s for each leg

Piriformis SMR: Hold on tender spots for 30s each leg

Afghan Squat Challenge: Max hold for time

Single Leg Glute Bridge: Max hold for time

Squat Test: Retest: 10 reps. Any change?

SCAN THIS CODE AND GET:

MY INJURY PREVENTION GUIDE

16

DID THE ARMY BREAK YOUR BRAIN?

Ryan Carey

Getting Up To Speed

Mild Traumatic Brain Injuries (mTBI) are the dirty little secret of the Army, affecting many of us but rarely discussed. I don't want to scare you, but if you spent any time as an infantry soldier, gunner, trooper, or assaulter, you likely had some mTBI exposure.

These jobs are dangerous, and there's a lot of stuff that goes BANG!

Until I came across Ryan Carey and his work with the Concussion Legacy Foundation, I wasn't aware of the concussive forces I'd been exposed to, which likely caused some mild brain trauma. In this chapter, I want to highlight the need for greater awareness of mTBI and what you can do about it.

mTBIs are concussions, plain and simple. They're considered "mild" because you don't have a massive hole in your skull or cerebrospinal fluid leaking out of your eyes. But taking these injuries lightly is a mistake.

A concussion is defined not as a "brain bruise" but as a violent "coup-contre-coup" injury, meaning some torque is applied to the brain inside the skull, resulting in injury. Picture whiplash from a car accident, not a rock falling on your head. Once this injury occurs, electrolytes leak from your brain cells.

Concussive forces often cause the brain to shift slightly in the skull. This micro-injury is usually not noticeable. However, if numerous, persistent concussive exposures occur over years, the accumulation can lead to serious brain trauma and potentially deadly Chronic Traumatic Encephalopathy (CTE). According to Ryan, these exposures happen regularly. For instance, breaching involves placing explosive charges to create a hole in a wall, a prime example of concussive shock that can cause an mTBI. Hard landings while parachuting, standing next to an artillery round going off, or, in my case, being near a Leopard 2 tank's main gun (which made me let out a primal roar but left my head feeling funny afterward) are all examples.

I briefly discussed concussions with Dallas Alexander, a retired JTF2 sniper. He said most assaulters would have thousands of jumps and would be exposed weekly to concussive forces during training.

> "It's the breachers that really started thinking about this as a problem because when they started teaching breaching, obviously, they started fine. Then they tried to find out, how close can we be to this blast." - Ryan Carey

The Concussion Legacy Foundation and their Operation Brain Health are leading the charge in Canada to raise awareness about mTBIs and CTE within the CAF community. Ryan Carey, their spokesman and a CAF veteran, grew up in a tough, country environment where he learned the value of hard work and perseverance. He excelled in football from a young age, eventually playing for a semi-pro team at 17, a university team, and then being drafted into the Canadian Football League. After playing for Winnipeg and Saskatchewan, Ryan volunteered to join the infantry with the Royal Canadian Regiment and went head-on into some of the fiercest fighting since Korea.

So, picture this: a former NFL player, Dave Duerson, starts investigating head injuries in football after experiencing the fallout himself. This quest led to holding the NFL accountable and a big win for change—limited contact during NFL practices, concussion protocols, and the admission that the league knew the damage it was doing to its players but didn't act on it sooner.

> "Playing in the NFL increases your likelihood of getting some type of neurological disorder like Parkinson's by 30%." - Ryan Carey

Who knew that NFL players and former soldiers would join forces in the fight against head injuries? Ryan Carey's efforts with Project Enlist are rallying troops to pledge their brains for research and giving veterans the support they deserve. According to Ryan:

> "Almost 70% of the initial brains pledged by soldiers showed signs of CTE." - Ryan Carey

My Experience

I spent a lot of time studying mTBIs during my master's research project and developed a concussion protocol for the high school where I worked. The reason a protocol is necessary for teenagers is the same reason adults need one: mitigating the damage from concussions can save lives.

I can't count how many exposures I've had, from running grenade ranges, claymore ranges, being next to a Leopard tank firing its main gun, 84mm ranges, falls, and fist fights. When you add it up, it makes sense that there might be room for concern, and I wasn't exposed nearly as much as someone in a special forces unit like Dallas or on the football field like Ryan.

Harden Up

Once we raise awareness about mTBIs, proper treatment can be implemented at all levels. The troubling issue is that some individuals diagnosed with psychological issues, such as PTSD, may actually be experiencing post-concussion syndrome.

Until further research is done, these numbers remain unclear. Read the next chapter (Removing the D from PTSD) for more interesting insights.

If you feel like you may have post-concussion syndrome and want to know more, head to the Concussion Legacy Foundation's Project Enlist website for more information.

Harden up.

17

REMOVING THE "D" FROM PTSD

Tom & Jen Satterly

Getting Up To Speed

Tom and Jen Satterly are doing incredible work through their All Secure Foundation. They're on a mission to help special forces warriors heal from psychological wounds, promoting the idea that Post Traumatic Stress isn't a disorder but a call to heal.

The current model for treating military personnel diagnosed with PTSD often involves removing them from their unit, isolating them at home, providing psychotherapy, and prescribing SSRIs. If these treatments are deemed ineffective, veterans may find themselves passed on to Veterans Affairs, facing more therapy and medications until they either find a better solution or give up.

Tom and Jen are developing an alternative path.

Tom is a former Delta Force Command Sergeant Major. To put that in context, he's a serious bad-ass, with his first combat experience being in Mogadishu, Somalia—the infamous "Black Hawk Down" incident that inspired the Ridley Scott movie. After his service, Tom reached a low point where he contemplated suicide but was saved by a call from Jen. He has since found a path to healing and now shares this journey to help others like him.

The All Secure Foundation is dedicated to supporting military families dealing with post-traumatic stress. Founded by the Satterlys, this organization embodies empathy, resilience, and understanding. By sharing their stories and offering unwavering support, they provide a lifeline for those navigating the complexities of post-traumatic stress.

Tom and Jen emphasize the importance of treating war trauma as a valid injury that requires medical attention, just like a physical wound. They discuss the use of the stellate ganglion block shot (SGB) to help alleviate the fight, flight, or freeze response associated with PTS. Their journey includes in-depth brain scans, revealing abnormalities and suggesting non-prescription treatments and hyperbaric oxygen therapy. Jen highlights the importance of brain scans, noting that trauma is trauma, regardless of its source.

> "I learned about the suicide epidemic at that time, which, honestly, I thought was not true. I didn't think it was accurate, and it isn't accurate. It's much higher than 22 a day. It's probably closer to 38 a day." - Jen Satterly

My Experience

The fact that I'm writing this book and you're reading it is pretty unbelievable. My life was in a bad place in 2019. After returning from Afghanistan, I quickly transitioned to teaching high school science to large classes of unruly teenagers. I remember breaking down in tears in my parent's basement because I didn't have a place to live yet. I felt immense anger and frustration, often struggling to control my emotions.

To cope, I drowned myself in work, taking on every extra task I could at my new school. I coached, ran clubs, competed in Spartan Races and CrossFit, and started a master's program at night—all while being a new dad with a new house.

A few years later, I was unemployed, recently released from the Army, and found myself crying after dropping my kids off at school. I wondered if this was the end of the road.

Thankfully, a motivational YouTube video by Jocko Willink caught my attention. I began listening to it daily, started getting up early, working out, writing, and building a small business. Eventually, I created my podcast. I also sought therapy and found support organizations that helped. Today, I'm in a much better place and can attest to Tom and Jen's belief that PTSD is not a permanent condition. It's not a disorder; it's a normal response to trauma that forces change.

Harden Up

The first step in recovery, if you're suffering from PTS, is to admit you need help. That was my initial hurdle. I was too proud to accept my disability award and even declined nearly two hundred thousand dollars, telling them I didn't want their money.

When it became clear that my world was crashing, I decided to attend the Veteran Transition Network program in Canada. Like the All Secure Foundation, the goal was to address the root of my trauma. You can't avoid it; you have to confront it, or it will never go away.

PTS is a complex issue, and I can't pretend to know what you're going through. However, I can offer this piece of advice: you are worth more to everyone around you alive, and people will be honored to help you get better, not burdened by it. If this book can help in any capacity, my hope is that it prevents at least one fellow warrior from taking their own life.

Harden up.

18

HEALING WITH PSYCHEDELICS

Carlos Duran & Ryan Carey

Getting Up To Speed

I never paid much attention to psychedelics. My impression from high school was that they were for stoners and dropouts, so I never took them seriously. It's funny how perspectives change as you get older. I had the pleasure of chatting with Carlos Duran and Ryan Carey about their veteran plant-medicine retreat called Operation Purify.

They take veterans from around the world to Colombia to heal through ayahuasca ceremonies. Initially, I thought this was some wild hippie stuff, but after hearing Ryan's experience, I realized there was merit to it.

Ayahuasca, psilocybin, ketamine, and cannabis are becoming

prevalent in the veteran community, and it's not by coincidence. Plant medicine has been around since the dawn of time, used in almost every culture, except ours, to heal from traumatic events and gain clarity on one's path forward.

Ayahuasca is a plant, specifically a root, found in regions like Colombia. It's boiled and consumed under the guidance of a "medicine man." Chemically, ayahuasca contains DMT, which allows the brain and central nervous system to process events from a completely different perspective. DMT has been called the "businessman's trip," and while it's naturally produced in the human body, ayahuasca provides a mega dose. Users report changes in perception, seeing geometric shapes, experiencing visions of past lives, or reliving traumas. The stories from veterans who have taken this medicine are some of the wildest I've heard. In an episode I did with Toby Miller, he described seeing his entire central nervous system being rewired.

Carlos emphasizes that ayahuasca won't have any effect if you don't let go and let it work. The program he's helped create isn't just a few days of tripping in the jungle; it requires preparation. Participants must start working out, stick to a schedule, and clean up their diet as part of respecting themselves and nature.

This aligns with a stoic quote:

> "What disgrace it is for a man to grow old without ever seeing the beauty and strength of which his body is capable." — Socrates

Carlos has great respect for the veteran community, saying:

> "Veterans give up their minds, bodies, and souls to protect their country." — Carlos Duran

This often results in tremendous trauma that needs to be resolved. Both Ryan and Carlos recognize that the modern medical approach of therapy and pharmaceuticals often only treats the symptoms, not the root causes of trauma, as ayahuasca does. This has been a fundamental criticism of modern medicine as well. For example, Toby Miller went from taking twenty-six medications to just one after drinking ayahuasca.

My Experience

In 2022, I went to Las Vegas to make business contacts and connect with the broader veteran business community at the Military Influencer Conference. I didn't expect the numerous conversations I'd have with fellow veterans about their "psychedelic" experiences healing from 20 years of war.

Ranger officers who had returned home and struggled with heroin addiction were now clean and thriving, and soldiers were no longer experiencing chronic pain. The list goes on. So, when I returned home, I decided to try it. I didn't go all-in; I ordered some microdose psilocybin capsules and gave them a try, intending to be honest with myself.

Well, I definitely became honest with myself. That night, I told my wife that I didn't feel connected to her at all. It had been bothering me for years, but I never had the courage to be honest with her. This conversation led to the worst event of my life: my wife and I separated a few months later. But there's a happy ending.

Nearly six months passed where I lived alone, explored deeper parts of myself, and continued microdosing. I realized I had a lot to unpack, and it felt like layers of heavy tarps were being lifted off me. It was hell—I cried myself to sleep most nights and wept harder than ever before. But there was a catharsis in all of this.

It allowed me to truly be myself again, take control of my life, and be a better man to my wife and children. Ultimately, this brought us back together, and I know psychedelics played an important role.

Harden Up

I can't say enough good things about Operation Purify, even though I haven't participated yet. I know I will, and I can see the impact it's already having in the veteran community, connecting people and changing lives. To learn more, reach out to them through their website and speak with Ryan or a team member to see if it's the right fit for you.

Harden up.

19

BREATHE MOTHER FUCKER

Brandon Powell

Getting Up To Speed

When I first saw Wim Hof plunging under the freezing waters of the Arctic and running up the Himalayas in shorts and nothing else, I thought, "What kind of gimmicky shit is this?"

I couldn't wrap my head around a human being able to do these things, so I dismissed it as nonsense. But curiosity got the better of me, and I found myself drawn back into Wim Hof's world. This time, it was through his Netflix documentary, The Iceman.

It turns out, this guy is a pure savage and has done more for the science of physiology in the last decade than most people, in my opinion. That's when I started paying attention and practicing his methods.

I had Brandon Powell on the show to chat about the Wim Hof Method since he's one of the OG coaches who has worked with Wim from the beginning. The essentials of the method are holotropic breathing and cold exposure. Essentially, it's about breathing deeply in a rhythmic pattern and then exposing yourself to cold water. According to Wim, the point of all this is to unlock the inner cellular machinery we all have, to manage stress, and to become a walking, healing machine.

Breathwork

Brandon breaks down how breathwork is the gateway to controlling your mind. For your logic center, or prefrontal cortex, to work effectively, you need to bring in plenty of oxygen and expel lots of carbon dioxide. For combat arms types, we did "box breathing" to "scan and breathe" after a firefight or clearing a room. This technique helps shift us from the "reptilian" fight-or-flight brain back to a thinking and reasoning state, regaining our senses and fine motor skills.

Holotropic breathing allows for deep relaxation, and part of this method includes practicing a breath hold. Interestingly, this hold is done after exhaling rather than inhaling.

Here's an example:

Fully in, fully out.

Fully in, fully out.

Fully in, fully out, and on your exhale, hold your breath for 1 minute.

If you feel the urge to breathe before the minute is up, that's okay.

Fully in and hold for 15 seconds.

Typically, you'd do 30 rounds of inhale/exhale before the breath hold. I've done up to five rounds and managed to hold my breath for over 3 minutes! Insane.

IMPORTANT: Don't do this type of breathwork in water, standing, or driving. Make sure you're sitting or lying down because fainting can happen.

Cold Plunges

Hopping into a cold tank or blasting yourself with cold water isn't pleasant, and that's the point. Like many concepts in this book, exposing yourself to the cold produces hormetic stress, a beneficial stress that stimulates a compensatory response. This response includes increased mitochondrial density through the activation of cold shock proteins. According to Brandon, regular cold exposure decreases your shiver response and makes you more resilient to cold—useful knowledge for Canadians.

What happens is that white fat, the kind that jiggles around our bellies, is transformed into brown fat. Brown fat is what babies have to keep themselves warm since they haven't developed a shivering reflex yet. Cool, right?

Brandon suggests starting with water around 55°F (about 10°C). Finish off your warm shower with a 15-second cold blast and gradually extend it. It sucks but is worth it. Trust me. After a week or so, lower the water temperature further or start immersing yourself in cold water for longer periods.

Beyond the physical benefits, exposure to cold has been shown to dramatically increase dopamine levels for hours afterward, more so than cocaine in terms of its long-lasting effects. Imagine combining that with the sensation of getting into a cold tank!

As Wim and Brandon say, "Get High Off Your Own Supply."

My Experience

When I was a kid, they used to call me "Dave The Polar Bear Morrow." My friends even made up a song for me. They claimed that my ability to last so long in our freezing cold pool was because I had more blubber on me, like a polar bear, and that's why they couldn't stand being in the water as long as I could.

Well, the joke's on them now. I'm a cold plunging, brown fat-producing, dopamine-crushing machine.

All jokes aside, I've found that getting into a cold tank brings a ton of focus back to my body and pulls me out of my head—a necessary shock when hopping into 2-degree water. This is where I think our current healthcare approach to mental health misses the mark. Cold plunging, BJJ, and hard workouts are all variations of the same principle: we need to get out of our heads and into our bodies. We need to provide "space" for our minds to heal. I guarantee that once you hit 2-degree water, the last thing you're thinking about is your trauma. Do this enough times, and you begin to train a new pattern. New neural pathways form, and you become significantly more resilient to stress.

Harden Up

Taking action on the Wim Hof Method is easy. There are loads of free, guided videos on YouTube—that's how I got started. You can then progress to Wim's app. If you'd like the full experience, I highly recommend reaching out to a coach like Brandon to take you to the next level and dive deep into your breathing and cold plunge practices.

The important thing is to take action now. Don't wait till tomorrow. Do a guided breathing session and blast yourself with cold water during your next shower. As always, this isn't a magic bullet, and results take time, but if you stick with it, you'll notice massive improvements in your mental and physical health.

Harden up and Breathe, Mother Fucker!

CONCLUSION - PUTTING IT ALL TOGETHER

The key to putting all this knowledge together and becoming harder to kill is understanding that you won't see massive changes overnight. Patience is crucial. Next, start reading. No one knows your body better than you do. No athletic therapist or doctor can "fix" you; that's your responsibility.

After reading this book, you should definitely pick up *The Nimble Warrior*, Canada's number one book on mobility for soldiers and first responders (shameless plug). I've also provided a list of books by all the experts I've interviewed at the end of this chapter.

When it comes to improving your fitness, especially strength, don't get bogged down by details like what gear to use or which exercise to do. At the end of the day, you need to struggle against something that requires you to use a significant amount of your musculature to push, press, or pull something regularly.

Start with the minimum effective dose concept. Do one day each week with 5 sets of 5 reps of something that's heavy as hell for you. You can use a variety of things. Next, set yourself up to win. Make it almost impossible to fail at your daily fitness habit. For example, I have a 5-push-ups-a-day streak that's been going on for years. Pick what works best for you and stick with it.

Set Up Your Streak

It's time to set up a streak or series of streaks. A streak is a concept I learned from James Clear's book, *Atomic Habits.* If you haven't read it, do so right after you finish this book. If you want to change your life, you need to set up a winning streak system for yourself. The chances of success increase significantly with this approach. I simply mark it down on a habit tracker sheet I made. Every time I complete a habit, I check it off. I do this with Wim Hof breathing.

You can find and download my habit tracker in my Veterans Getting Fit AF community or use the link in the References section.

Establish Your New Training Paradigm

The pandemic has taught us that we can't rely solely on gyms to maintain our fitness. Fitness is everywhere, and we need to embrace it.

I learned the concept of the austere gym from CrossFit.com and lived it while deployed to Afghanistan. We had some barbells and plates, but I also used picnic tables, ammo cans, jerry cans, and low concrete walls as training implements.

SCAN THIS CODE AND JOIN:

MY VETS GETTING FIT AF COMMUNITY

Make fitness as important as going to work or taking care of your kids.

The H.A.R.D. To Kill Protocol

I've been inspired by every one of the guests on my podcast to become a better human being. Each guest featured in these chapters is doing incredible work to help others achieve greatness. But reading about all this alpha energy is useless if you don't put it into action.

That's why I've created the H.A.R.D. To Kill Protocol. This is a simple, day-by-day program you can follow at home to reset your mind, body, and soul so that you can become harder to kill. If you follow this protocol, you will lose fat, improve your strength, accomplish more with more energy, and be more present in your day-to-day life than you could have imagined.

Your H.A.R.D. To Kill Protocol Weekly Template

Use this weekly template to create your plan. Every week, there will be new things to add. Use the progressions and workouts I've created as your guide.

The Battle Plan

This is an everyday plan. Thirty days of hardening up—no excuses for birthdays or vacations. If you miss a day, you start again at day one. Now that we're all in agreement, let's get after it.

You can find guided videos and descriptions of all the workouts (WODs) listed below by heading to www.hardtokill.org.

Use the hashtag #hrd2kill during your hardening up and healing journey. This is just the tip of the iceberg. Once you're done with your 30-Day H.A.R.D. Routine, you can head to my merch store and pick up some exclusive, congratulatory merchandise at davemorrow.net/merch.

You've earned it.

Go Forth and Become Harder to Kill

WEEK 1 PLAN

DAILY NON-NEGOTIABLES

- 20 minutes of PT
- 1 cycle of breathwork or mindfulness practice
- 15 sec of cold shower or ice bath
- No cell phones 1 hr before bedtime
- Read a book for 20 minutes
- SMR for 10 mins watching TV
- Journal for 5 mins (Record your streaks)

TASKS FOR THE WEEK

Do this WOD twice during the week:

- 3 x 10-12 reps KB RDL
- 3 x 8-10 reps Poor man's HSC
- 50 air squats
- 30 sit-ups

WEEK 2 PLAN

DAILY NON-NEGOTIABLES

- 20 minutes of PT
- 1 cycle of breathwork or mindfulness practice
- 15 sec of cold shower or ice bath
- No cell phones 1 hr before bedtime
- Read a book for 20 minutes
- SMR for 10 mins watching TV
- Journal for 5 mins (Record your streaks)

TASKS FOR THE WEEK

Do this WOD twice during the week:
- 3 x 10-12 reps KB RDL
- 3 x 8-10 reps Poor man's HSC
- 50 air squats
- 30 sit-ups

Pick a combat sport and attend a class (preferably BJJ)

No snacks, eat 1g/lb of desired body weight of protein

146

WEEK 3 PLAN

DAILY NON-NEGOTIABLES

- 20 minutes of PT
- 1 cycle of breathwork or mindfulness practice
- 15 sec of cold shower or ice bath
- No cell phones 1 hr before bedtime
- Read a book for 20 minutes
- SMR for 10 mins watching TV
- Journal for 5 mins (Record your streaks)

TASKS FOR THE WEEK

Do this WOD twice during the week:

- 3 x 10-12 reps KB RDL
- 3 x 8-10 reps Poor man's HSC
- 60 air squats
- 40 sit-ups
- 60 push-ups

Pick a combat sport and attend a class (preferably BJJ)
No snacks, eat 1g/lb of desired body weight of protein
Remove all sugar from your diet

WEEK 4 PLAN

DAILY NON-NEGOTIABLES

- 20 minutes of PT
- 1 cycle of breathwork or mindfulness practice
- 15 sec of cold shower or ice bath
- No cell phones 1 hr before bedtime
- Read a book for 20 minutes
- SMR for 10 mins watching TV
- Journal for 5 mins (Record your streaks)

TASKS FOR THE WEEK

Do this WOD twice during the week:
- 3 x 10-12 reps KB RDL
- 3 x 8-10 reps Poor man's HSC
- 70 air squats
- 50 sit-ups
- 60 push-ups

Pick a combat sport and attend a class (preferably BJJ)
No snacks, eat 1g/lb of desired body weight of protein
Remove all sugar from your diet
Fast for 1 x 24hrs
Microdose psilocybin

The Final Task

Now, there's one more thing you must do: be an advocate for change. Reading this book isn't enough. Share it with a fellow veteran who needs a kick in the ass or a civilian who's just coasting through life. You'll help spread the message of this podcast, which is all about helping others learn how to not merely exist but thrive, so we can all be pillars of our communities.

I hope this book has inspired you and that you will take immediate action to become harder to kill. I'd love to hear about your journey, so please reach out to me on my socials.

Train Hard, Fight Easy.

REFERENCES

Introduction

Obesity rates - https://www.ncbi.nlm.nih.gov/pmc/articles/PMC7530827/

Mental health issues - https://www.ncbi.nlm.nih.gov/pmc/articles/PMC7530827/

Veteran suicide rates - https://www.military.com/daily-news/2021/06/21/9-11-suicide-has-claimed-four-times-more-military-lives-combat.html

Prepare Your Mind Like A Sniper

Carol Dweck, "Mindset." (https://amzn.to/3zqqvsR)

Operation Pegasus Jump. (https://operationpegasus.ca)

Change Your Story, Change Your Mind

Enlifted Coaching (https://enlifted.me/)

Don't Get Outflanked

Hal Hughes Counselling (https://www.halhughes.com/)

Men Are Dying For New Mental Health Approach

Dr. Robert Whitley, Men's Issues and Men's Mental Health: An Introductory Primer (https://amzn.to/3RSXmgi)

Warrior Adventures Canada (https://warrioradventures.ca/)

Irreverent Warriors (https://irreverentwarriors.com/)

Becoming Om (https://www.becomingom.com/)

Voluntold (https://www.voluntold.co/)

Addiction Can Ruin You

Dr. Robb Kelly, "Daddy, Daddy, Please Stop Drinking" (https://amzn.to/4cpyuVz)

Be Mindful Like a Navy SEAL

Jon Macaskill, "Unleashing Inner Strength: A Navy SEAL's Guide to Preparedness, Resilience, Grit, and Compassion Through Mindfulness" (https://amzn.to/4cNvO48)

Marcus Luttrell, "Lone Survivor The Eyewitness Account of Operation Redwing and the Lost Heroes of SEAL Team 10" (https://amzn.to/3RUxuAH)

The Lions Are Home From War

Stuart Scheller, "Crisis of Command: How We Lost Trust and Confidence in America's Generals and Politicians" (https://amzn.to/3XOjPPg)

Stop Eating Like A 10 Year Old

Ben Azadi, "Keto Flex: The 4 Secrets to Reduce Inflammation, Burn Fat & Reboot Your Metabolism" (https://amzn.to/3XQE8M6)

Fasting For Longevity

Cynthia Thurlow, "Fasting For Longevity" (https://amzn.to/4bLkswF)

Cholesterol Won't Kill You. Poor Metabolic Health Will

Dr. Philip Ovadia, "Stay Off My Operating Table" (https://amzn.to/4bxRiAR)

BJJ Will Save Us All

Dr. Gino Collura, "Seven Layers of Successful Relationships" (https://amzn.to/3VOpvGp)

The Hard Truth About Erectile Dysfunction

Dr. Judson Brandeis, "The 21st Century Man: Advice From 50 Top Doctors and Men's Health Experts so You Can Feel Great, Look Good and Have Better Sex"

FirmTech Ring: https://myfirmtech.com/h2kpod (Code: DMORROW)

P-Long study: https://p-long.com/wp-content/uploads/2022/10/P-Long_Study_Abstract.pdf

Destroy Dad Bod

Jason Khalipa, "As Many Reps As Possible" (https://amzn.to/3RTiIu0)

Sleep or Die

Dr. Kirk Parsley, "Sleep to Win: How Navy SEALs and Other High Performers Stay on Top." (https://amzn.to/3RPYaTi)

Control Your Pain and Stay Supple

Dr. Kelly Starrett, "Becoming a Supple Leopard 2nd Edition: The Ultimate Guide to Resolving Pain, Preventing Injury, and Optimizing Athletic Performance" (https://amzn.to/4bsrp5n)

Dr. Kelly Starrett, "Deskbound: Standing Up to a Sitting World" (https://amzn.to/3zuD4TY)

Dr. Kelly Starrett, "Ready to Run: Unlocking Your Potential to Run Naturally" (https://amzn.to/4btZfHg)

Dave Morrow, "The Nimble Warrior" (https://amzn.to/41UpZO0)

Did The Army Break Your Brain?

The Concussion Legacy Foundation (https://www.concussionfoundation.ca/)

Removing the "D" From PTSD

Tom Satterly, "All Secure: A Special Operations Soldier's Fight to Survive on the Battlefield and the Homefront" (https://amzn.to/3RROhnO)

All Secure Foundation (https://www.allsecurefoundation.org/)

Healing With Psychedelics

Operation Purify (https://operationpurify.com/)

Breathe Mother F*cker

Wim Hoff, "The Wim Hof Method: Activate Your Full Human Potential" (https://amzn.to/3zw29Ow)

Brandon Powell Coaching (https://www.wimhofmethod.com/instructors/brandonpowell)

Putting It All Together

Habit Tracker (https://docs.google.com/document/d/1JDDb26KmevR7jOE-pfwMc36JjaG_Z3U7AjVroQi9IKM/edit?usp=sharing)

Veterans Getting Fit AF Community (https://www.skool.com/dave-morrow-personal-training/about)

Hard To Kill Website (https://hardtokill.org/)

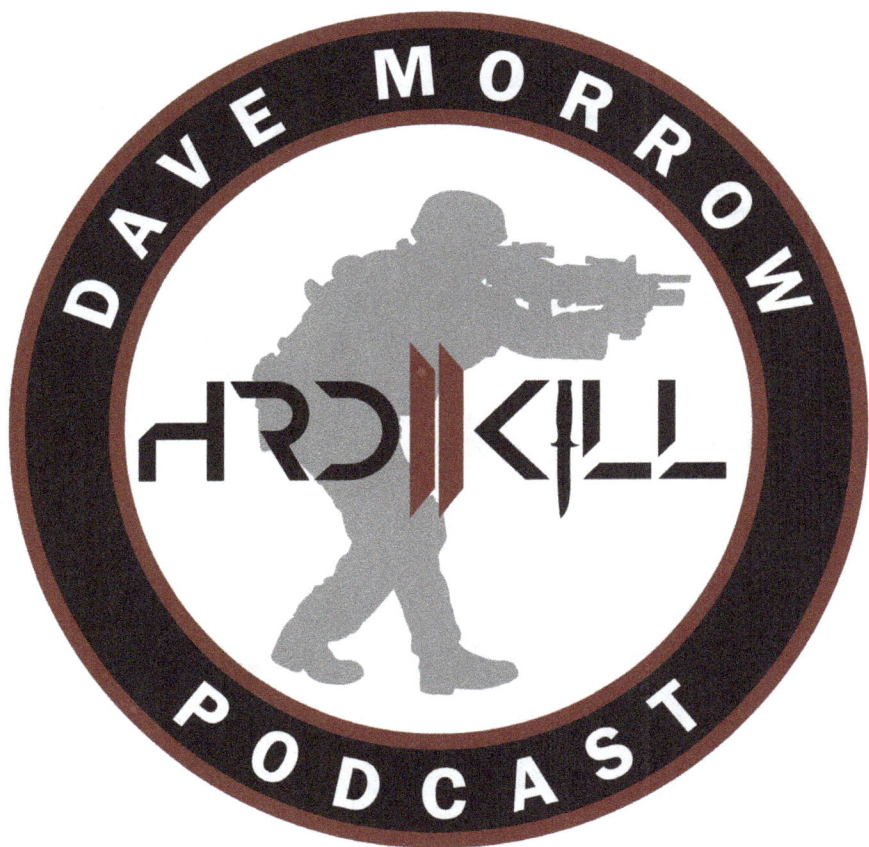

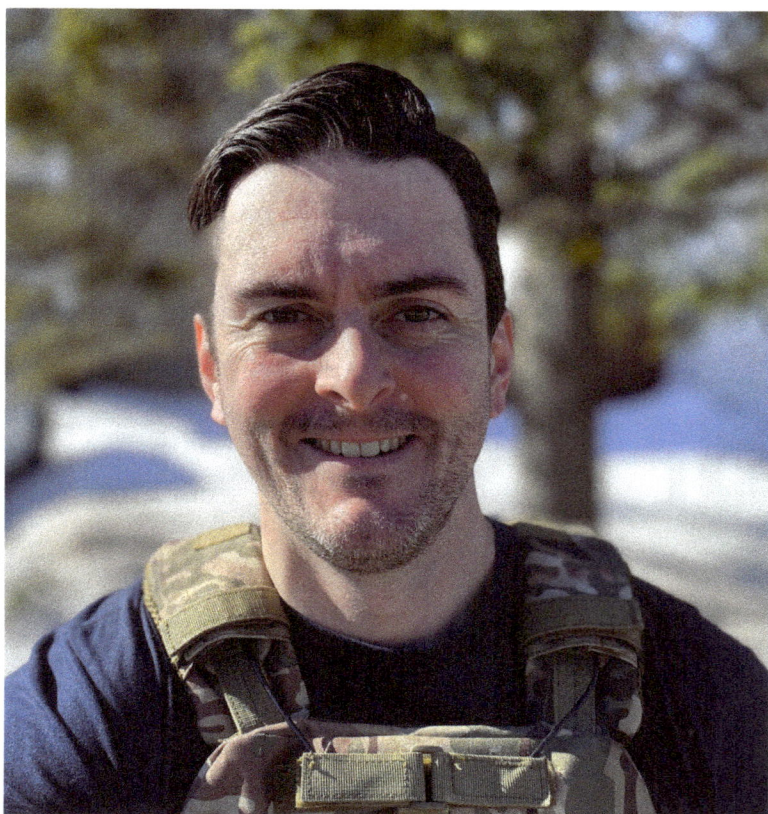

ABOUT THE AUTHOR

I grew up in the Army. It taught me the valuable lessons of grueling hard work, the importance of a solid team, how to get shit done when the chips are down and how to motivate people in the worst of situations. Ever since I was a kid growing up in the suburbs of Montreal, I had visions of being a soldier like my grandpa. Before deploying to Afghanistan in 2010, I had the bright idea of becoming a chemist and received biochemistry and teaching degrees from McGill University. I taught highschool math and science for nearly ten years before embarking on my current path of helping the veteran community improve their health and fitness.

Now, when I'm not podcasting, working out or coaching fellow veterans, I'm playing with my two high-energy children or planning our next, big family trip.

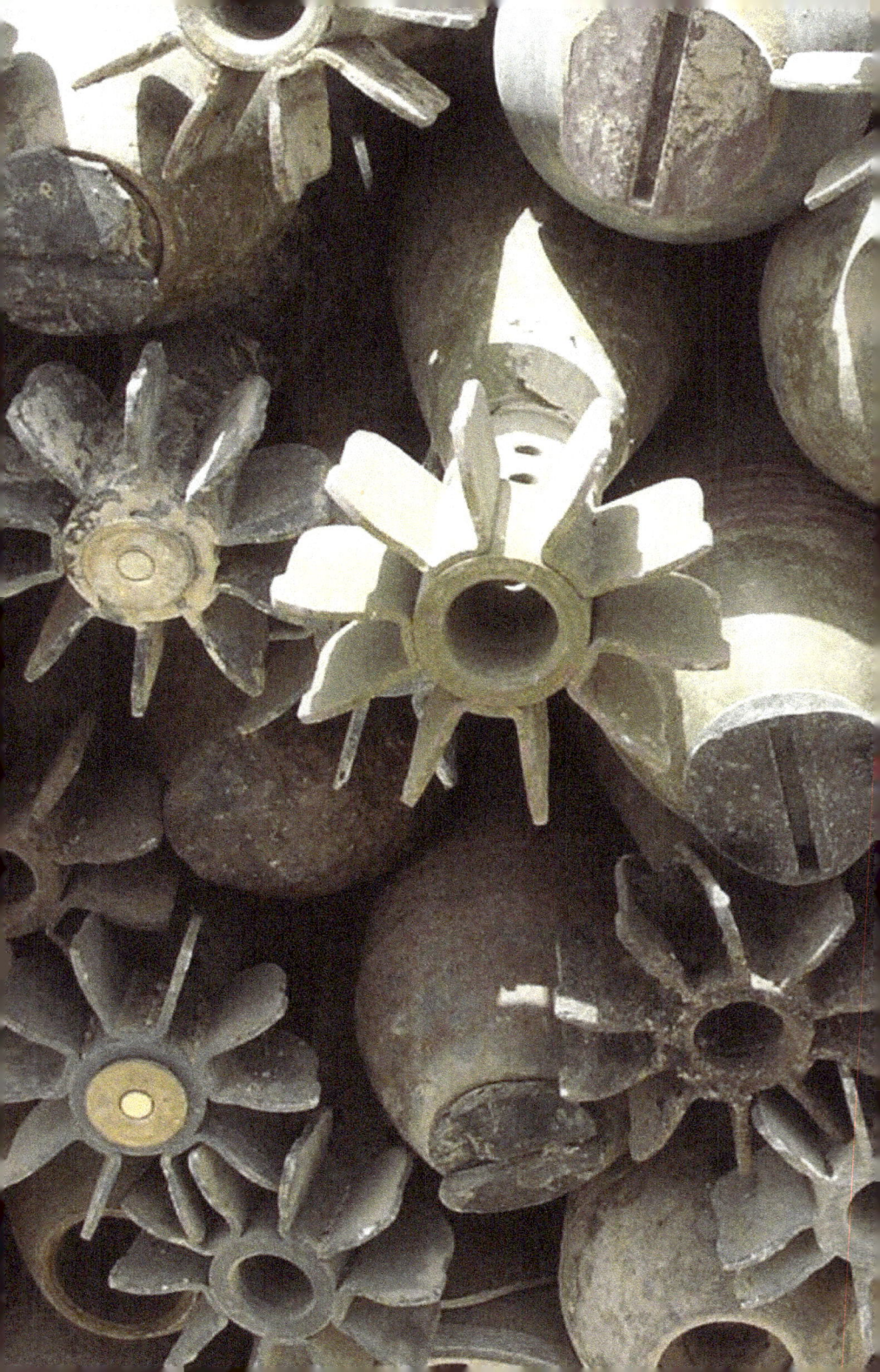

DOUBLE‡DAGGER
— www.doubledagger.ca —

DOUBLE DAGGER BOOKS is Canada's only military-focused publisher. Conflict and warfare have shaped human history since before we began to record it. The earliest stories that we know of, passed on as oral tradition, speak of war, and more importantly, the essential elements of the human condition that are revealed under its pressure.

We are dedicated to publishing material that, while rooted in conflict, transcend the idea of "war" as merely a genre. Fiction, non-fiction, and stuff that defies categorization, we want to read it all.

Because if you want peace, study war.

If you loved this book, you could help another veteran unlock their health potential by leaving a review on Amazon or Goodreads.